NINTH EDITION

WEST'S PULMONARY PATHOPHYSIOLOGY

THE ESSENTIALS

John B. West, MD, PhD

Distinguished Professor of Medicine and Physiology
University of California, San Diego
School of Medicine
San Diego, California

Andrew M. Luks, MD

Professor of Medicine
University of Washington School of Medicine
Seattle, Washington

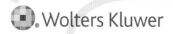 Wolters Kluwer

Philadelphia · Baltimore · New York · London
Buenos Aires · Hong Kong · Sydney · Tokyo

Acquisitions Editor: Crystal Taylor
Product Development Editor: Christine Fahey
Development Editor: Andrea Vosburgh
Editorial Coordinator: Lauren Pecarich
Editorial Assistant: Brooks Phelps
Marketing Manager: Michael McMahon
Production Project Manager: Bridgett Dougherty
Design Coordinator: Holly McLaughlin
Manufacturing Coordinator: Margie Orzech
Prepress Vendor: SPi Global

Ninth Edition

Copyright © 2017 Wolters Kluwer

First Edition, 1977
Second Edition, 1982
Third Edition, 1987
Fourth Edition, 1992
Fifth Edition, 1998
Sixth Edition, 2003
Seventh Edition, 2008
Eighth Edition, 2013

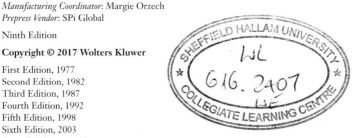

9 8 7 6 5 4 3 2 1

Printed in China

Library of Congress Cataloging-in-Publication Data
Names: West, John B. (John Burnard), author. | Luks, Andrew, author. | Complemented by (expression): West, John B. (John Burnard). West's respiratory physiology. 10th edition.
Title: West's pulmonary pathophysiology : the essentials / John B. West, Andrew M. Luks.
Other titles: Pulmonary pathophysiology
Description: Ninth edition. | Philadelphia : Wolters Kluwer, [2017] | Preceded by Pulmonary pathophysiology : the essentials / John B. West. 8th ed. 2013. | Complemented by West's respiratory physiology / John B. West, Andrew M. Luks. 10th ed. 2016. | Includes bibliographical references and index.
Identifiers: LCCN 2016046551 | ISBN 9781496339447
Subjects: | MESH: Lung Diseases—physiopathology | Respiratory Function Tests | Lung—pathology
Classification: LCC RC711 | NLM WF 600 | DDC 616.2/407—dc23 LC record available at https://lccn.loc.gov/2016046551

To R.B.W.

—*John B. West*

To all my students.

—*Andrew M. Luks*

REVIEWERS

Dionisio Acosta
San Juan Bautista School of Medicine
Class of 2017
Caguas, Puerto Rico

Rasha Ahmed
Western University of Health Sciences
Class of 2017
Pomona, California

Sharde Chambers
Rowan University School of Osteopathic Medicine
Class of 2017
Stratford, New Jersey

Sarah Corral
Oakland University William Beaumont School of Medicine
Class of 2018
Rochester, Michigan

Jay Dean, PhD
Professor
Department of Molecular Pharmacology and Physiology
University of South Florida Morsani College of Medicine
Tampa, Florida

Gliceida M. Galarza Fortuna
Universidad Iberoamericana
Class of 2017
Mexico City, Mexico

Kelsi Hirai
University of Hawaii John A Burns School of Medicine
Class of 2017
Honolulu, Hawaii

Justin Lytle
Touro University Nevada
Class of 2018
Henderson, Nevada

Michael P. Madaio
University of New England College of Osteopathic Medicine
Class of 2018
Biddeford, Maine

Niral Patel
Lake Erie College of Osteopathic Medicine–Bradenton Campus
Class of 2018
Bradenton, Florida

Robert R. Preston, PhD
Formerly Associate Professor
Department of Pharmacology and Physiology
Drexel University College of Medicine
Philadelphia, Pennsylvania

Sakeina Wilson
Rowan School of Osteopathic Medicine
Class of 2017
Stratford, New Jersey

Eric Woods
Icahn School of Medicine at Mount Sinai
Class of 2017
New York, New York

PREFACE

This book is a companion to *West's Respiratory Physiology, 10th edition* (Wolters Kluwer, 2016) and is about the function of the diseased lung as opposed to the normal lung. It was first published 40 years ago and has therefore served several generations of students. It has been translated into a number of languages. This ninth edition has many extensive changes. The most significant is that Andrew M. Luks, MD, has become a coauthor. Dr. Luks obtained his MD at the School of Medicine, University of California San Diego, and was therefore exposed to much of this material as a medical student. He is now on the faculty at the University of Washington School of Medicine where he enjoys a reputation as an excellent teacher. As he was when he became a coauthor on the 10th edition of *West's Respiratory Physiology*, he has been responsible for many of the important changes in this new edition, particularly the clinical vignettes, many new multiple choice questions, and a number of new illustrations.

Each chapter now has a clinical vignette that emphasizes how the pathophysiology described in the chapter is used in the practice of clinical medicine. At the end of the vignette are several questions and answers to these are in an appendix. Another addition is over 30 new multiple choice questions in the format used by the USMLE. The stems of these questions have a clinical orientation, and their purpose is to test the broader understanding of a topic rather than a simple factual recall. The illustrative material in the book has been considerably expanded with eight new radiographs and CT images as well as color histopathologic sections graciously provided to us by Corinne Fligner, MD, from the University of Washington School of Medicine and Edward Klatt, MD, from Mercer University School of Medicine. The text of the book has been updated in many areas particularly in the sections dealing with modern therapy. Another new development has been the production of seven 50-minute video lectures based on the book. These are freely available on YouTube and have proved to be very popular.

As a result of all these innovations, the length of the book has been increased, but its primary purpose has not changed. As before, it serves as an introductory text for medical students in their second and subsequent years. However, a concise, amply illustrated account of respiratory function in disease will prove useful to the increasingly large number of physicians (such as anesthesiologists and cardiologists) and other medical personnel (including intensive care nurses and respiratory therapists) who come into contact with respiratory patients.

The authors are grateful for any comments on the selection of material or any factual errors. We will respond to any e-mails on these subjects.

John B. West, jwest@ucsd.edu

Andrew M. Luks, aluks@u.washington.edu

CONTENTS

Reviewers vi
Preface viii

PART ONE Lung Function Tests and What They Mean

CHAPTER 1 VENTILATION 3

CHAPTER 2 GAS EXCHANGE 20

CHAPTER 3 OTHER TESTS 44

PART TWO Function of the Diseased Lung

CHAPTER 4 OBSTRUCTIVE DISEASES 61

CHAPTER 5 RESTRICTIVE DISEASES 96

CHAPTER 6 VASCULAR DISEASES 120

CHAPTER 7 ENVIRONMENTAL, NEOPLASTIC,
AND INFECTIOUS DISEASES 146

PART THREE Function of the Failing Lung

CHAPTER 8 RESPIRATORY FAILURE 173

CHAPTER 9 OXYGEN THERAPY 189

CHAPTER 10 MECHANICAL VENTILATION 205

APPENDIX A—Symbols, Units, and Normal Values 219
APPENDIX B—Further Reading 222
APPENDIX C—Answers to the End-of-Chapter Questions 223
APPENDIX D—Answers to Questions in Clinical Vignettes 236

Index 243

LUNG FUNCTION TESTS AND WHAT THEY MEAN

1 ■ **Ventilation**

2 ■ **Gas Exchange**

3 ■ **Other Tests**

We learn how diseased lungs work by doing pulmonary function tests. Accordingly, Part One is devoted to a description of the most important tests and their interpretation. It is assumed that the reader is familiar with the basic physiology of the lung as contained in the companion volume, West JB, Luks AM. *West's Respiratory Physiology: The Essentials*. 10th ed. Philadelphia, PA: Wolters Kluwer, 2016.

VENTILATION

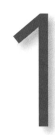

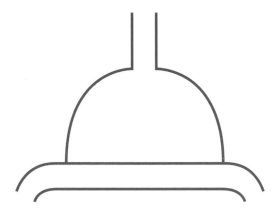

- **Tests of Ventilatory Capacity**
  Forced Expiratory Volume
  Forced Expiratory Flow
  Interpretation of Tests of Forced
    Expiration
  Expiratory Flow–Volume Curve
  Partitioning of Flow Resistance
    from the Flow–Volume Curve
  Maximum Flows from the Flow–
    Volume Curve
  Peak Expiratory Flow Rate
  Inspiratory Flow–Volume Curve

- **Tests of Uneven Ventilation**
  Single-Breath Nitrogen Test
  Closing Volume
  Other Tests of Uneven
    Ventilation
  Tests of Early Airway Disease

The simplest test of lung function is a forced expiration. It is also one of the most informative tests, and it requires minimal equipment and trivial calculations. The majority of patients with lung disease have an abnormal forced expiration volume, and, very often, the information obtained from this test is useful in their management. The test has great utility in primary care clinics when patients present for evaluation of chronic dyspnea. For example, it can be valuable in detecting asthma and chronic obstructive pulmonary diseases, extremely common and important conditions. This chapter also discusses a simple test of uneven ventilation.

TESTS OF VENTILATORY CAPACITY

Forced Expiratory Volume

The *forced expiratory volume* (FEV_1) is the volume of gas exhaled in *1 second* by a forced expiration from full inspiration. The *vital capacity* is the *total* volume of gas that can be exhaled after a full inspiration.

The simple, classic way of making these measurements is shown in **Figure 1.1**. The patient is comfortably seated in front of a spirometer having a low resistance. He or she breathes in maximally and then exhales as hard and as far as possible. As the spirometer bell moves up, the kymograph pen moves down, thus indicating the expired volume against time. The water-filled spirometer shown in Figure 1.1 is now seldom used and has been replaced by electronic spirometers that often provide a graph to be filed with the patient's chart or in the patient's electronic medical record.

Figure 1.2A shows a normal tracing. The volume exhaled in 1 second was 4.0 liters, and the total volume exhaled was 5.0 liters. These two volumes are therefore the forced expiratory volume in 1 second (FEV_1) and the vital capacity, respectively. The vital capacity measured with a forced expiration may be less than that measured with a slower exhalation, so that the term *forced vital capacity* (FVC) is generally used.

These values are reported both as absolute values and as a percentage of what one would predict for an individual of the same age, gender, and height.

The ratio of the FEV_1 to FVC (FEV_1/FVC) is also reported. The normal value is approximately 80% but decreases with age (see Appendix A for

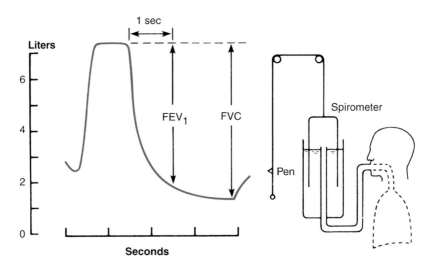

Figure 1.1. Measurement of forced expiratory volume (FEV_1) and forced vital capacity (FVC).

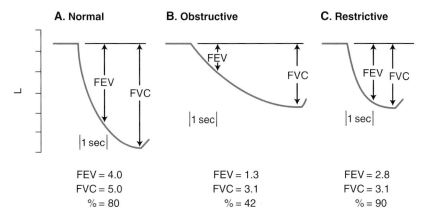

A. Normal   **B. Obstructive**   **C. Restrictive**

FEV = 4.0   FEV = 1.3   FEV = 2.8
FVC = 5.0   FVC = 3.1   FVC = 3.1
% = 80   % = 42   % = 90

Figure 1.2. **Normal, obstructive, and restrictive patterns of a forced expiration.**

normal values). Expert guidelines put forth by various organizations include more refined definitions for the lower limit of normal for the FEV_1/FVC ratio, but the 80% cutoff is a useful threshold for the beginning student.

The FEV can be measured over other times, such as 2 or 3 seconds, but the 1-second value is the most informative. When the subscript is omitted, the time is 1 second.

Figure 1.2B shows the type of tracing obtained from a patient with chronic obstructive pulmonary disease (COPD). Note that the rate at which the air was exhaled was much slower, so that only 1.3 liters were blown out in the first second. In addition, the total volume exhaled was only 3.1 liters. FEV_1/FVC was reduced to 42%. These figures are typical of an *obstructive* pattern.

Contrast this pattern with that of **Figure 1.2C**, which shows the type of tracing obtained from a patient with pulmonary fibrosis. Here, the vital capacity was reduced to 3.1 liters, but a large percentage (90%) was exhaled in the first second. These figures mean *restrictive* disease. Note that the specific numerical values in these examples have been inserted for illustrative purposes and will vary between patients, but the general pattern will remain the same between patients with each category of diseases.

The patient should loosen tight clothing, and the mouthpiece should be at a convenient height. One accepted procedure is to allow two practice blows and then record three good test breaths. The highest FEV_1 and FVC from these three breaths are then used. The volumes should be converted to body temperature and pressure (see Appendix A).

The test is often valuable in assessing the efficacy of bronchodilator drugs. If reversible airway obstruction is suspected, the test should be carried out before and after administering the drug (e.g., albuterol by nebulizer or metered-dose inhaler). Both the FEV_1 and FVC usually increase in a patient with bronchospasm.

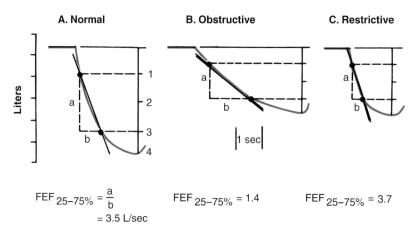

Figure 1.3. Calculation of forced expiratory flow (FEF$_{25-75\%}$) from a forced expiration.

FEV$_1$ and FVC

The 1-second forced expiratory volume together with the forced vital capacity is

• A simple test
• Often informative
• Abnormal in many patients with lung disease
• Often valuable in assessing the progress of disease

Forced Expiratory Flow

This index is calculated from a forced expiration, as shown in **Figure 1.3**. The middle half (by volume) of the total expiration is marked, and its duration is measured. The FEF$_{25-75\%}$ is the volume in liters divided by the time in seconds.

The correlation between FEF$_{25-75\%}$ and FEV$_1$ is generally close in patients with obstructive pulmonary disease. The changes in FEF$_{25-75\%}$ are often more striking, but the range of normal values is greater.

Interpretation of Tests of Forced Expiration

In some respects, the lungs and thorax can be regarded as a simple air pump **(Figure 1.4)**. The output of such a pump depends on the stroke volume, the resistance of the airways, and the force applied to the piston. The last factor is relatively unimportant in a forced expiration, as we shall presently see.

The *vital capacity* (or forced vital capacity) is a measure of the stroke volume, and any reduction of it affects the ventilatory capacity. Causes of stroke volume reduction include diseases of the thoracic cage, such as kyphoscoliosis,

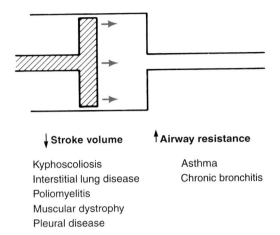

↓ **Stroke volume**   ↑ **Airway resistance**

Kyphoscoliosis   Asthma
Interstitial lung disease   Chronic bronchitis
Poliomyelitis
Muscular dystrophy
Pleural disease

Figure 1.4. Simple model of factors that may reduce the ventilatory capacity. The stroke volume may be reduced by diseases of the chest wall, lung parenchyma, respiratory muscles, and pleura. Airway resistance is increased in asthma and bronchitis.

ankylosing spondylitis, and acute injuries; diseases affecting the nerve supply to the respiratory muscles or the muscles themselves, such as poliomyelitis and muscular dystrophy; abnormalities of the pleural cavity, such as pneumothorax and pleural thickening; disease in the lung itself, such as fibrosis, which reduces its distensibility; space-occupying lesions, such as cysts; or an increased pulmonary blood volume, as in left heart failure. In addition, there are diseases of the airways that cause them to close prematurely during expiration, thus limiting the volume that can be exhaled. This occurs in asthma and chronic bronchitis.

The *forced expiratory volume* (and related indices such as the $FEF_{25-75\%}$) is affected by the airway resistance during forced expiration. Any increase in resistance reduces the ventilatory capacity. Causes include bronchoconstriction, as in asthma or following the inhalation of irritants such as cigarette smoke; structural changes in the airways, as in chronic bronchitis; obstructions within the airways, such as an inhaled foreign body or excess bronchial secretions; and destructive processes in the lung parenchyma that interfere with the radial traction that normally holds the airways open.

The simple model of Figure 1.4 introduces the factors limiting the ventilatory capacity of the diseased lung, but we need to refine the model to obtain a better understanding. For example, the airways are actually *inside*, not *outside*, the pump, as shown in Figure 1.4. Useful additional information comes from the flow–volume curve.

Expiratory Flow–Volume Curve

If we record flow rate and volume during a maximal forced expiration, we obtain a pattern like that shown in **Figure 1.5A**. A curious feature of the flow–volume curve is that it is virtually impossible to get outside it. For example,

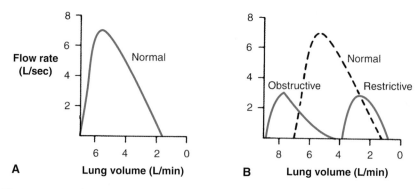

Figure 1.5. Expiratory flow–volume curves. A. Normal. **B.** Obstructive and restrictive patterns.

if we begin by exhaling slowly and then exert maximum effort, the flow rate increases to the envelope but not beyond. Clearly, something very powerful is limiting the maximum flow rate at a given volume. This factor is *dynamic compression of the airways.*

Figure 1.5B shows typical patterns found in obstructive and restrictive lung disease. In obstructive diseases, such as chronic bronchitis and emphysema, the maximal expiration typically begins and ends at abnormally high lung volumes, and the flow rates are much lower than normal. In addition, the curve may have a scooped-out appearance. By contrast, patients with restrictive disease, such as interstitial fibrosis, operate at low lung volumes. Their flow envelope is flattened compared with a normal curve, but if flow rate is related to lung volume, the flow is seen to be higher than normal (Figure 1.5B). Note that the figure shows absolute lung volumes, although these cannot be obtained from a forced expiration. They require an additional measurement of residual volume.

To understand these patterns, consider the pressures inside and outside the airways **(Figure 1.6)** (see *West's Respiratory Physiology: The Essentials.* 10th ed. p. 121). Before inspiration (A), the pressures in the mouth, airways, and alveoli are all atmospheric because there is no flow. Intrapleural pressure is, say, 5 cm H_2O below atmospheric pressure, and we assume that the same pressure exists outside the airways (although this is an oversimplification). Thus, the pressure difference expanding the airways is 5 cm H_2O. At the beginning of inspiration (B), all pressures fall and the pressure difference holding the airways open increases to 6 cm H_2O. At the end of inspiration (C), this pressure is 8 cm H_2O.

Early in a forced expiration (D), both intrapleural and alveolar pressures rise greatly. The pressure at some point in the airways increases, but not as much as does alveolar pressure because of the pressure drop caused by flow. Under these circumstances, we have a pressure difference of 11 cm H_2O, which tends to *close* the airways. Airway compression occurs, and now flow is determined by the difference between alveolar pressure and the pressure outside the airways

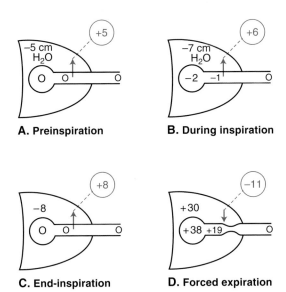

A. Preinspiration **B. During inspiration**

C. End-inspiration **D. Forced expiration**

Figure 1.6. Diagram to explain dynamic compression of the airways during a forced expiration (see text for details).

at the collapse point (Starling resistor effect). Note that this pressure difference (8 cm H_2O in D) is the static recoil pressure of the lung and it depends only on lung volume and compliance. It is *independent* of expiratory effort.

How then can we explain the abnormal patterns in Figure 1.5B? In the patient with chronic bronchitis and emphysema, the low flow rate in relation to lung volume is caused by several factors. There may be thickening of the walls of the airways and excessive secretions in the lumen because of bronchitis; both increase the flow resistance. The number of small airways may be reduced because of destruction of lung tissue. Also, the patient may have a reduced static recoil pressure (even though lung volume is greatly increased) because of breakdown of elastic alveolar walls. Finally, the normal support offered to the airways by the traction of the surrounding parenchyma is probably impaired because of loss of alveolar walls, and the airways therefore collapse more easily than they should. These factors are considered in more detail in Chapter 4.

Dynamic Compression of the Airways

- Limits flow rate during a forced expiration
- Causes flow to be independent of effort
- May limit flow during normal expiration in some patients with COPD
- Is a major factor limiting exercise in COPD

The patient with interstitial fibrosis has normal (or high) flow rates in relation to lung volume because the lung static recoil pressures are high and the caliber of the airways may be normal (or even increased) at a given lung volume. However, because of the greatly reduced compliance of the lung, volumes are very small, and absolute flow rates are therefore reduced. These changes are further discussed in Chapter 5.

This analysis shows that Figure 1.4 is a considerable oversimplification and that the FEV, which seems so straightforward at first, is affected both by the airways and by the lung parenchyma. Thus, the terms "obstructive" and "restrictive" conceal a good deal of pathophysiology.

Partitioning of Flow Resistance from the Flow–Volume Curve

When the airways collapse during a forced expiration, the flow rate is determined by the resistance of the airways up to the point of collapse **(Figure 1.7)**. Beyond this point, the resistance of the airways is immaterial. Collapse occurs at (or near) the point where the pressure inside the airways is equal to the intrapleural pressure (*equal pressure point*). This is believed to be in the vicinity of the lobar bronchi early in a forced expiration. However, as lung volume reduces and the airways narrow, their resistance increases. As a result, pressure is lost more rapidly, and the collapse point moves into more distal airways. Thus, late in forced expiration, flow is increasingly determined by the properties of the small distal peripheral airways.

These peripheral airways (say, less than 2 mm in diameter) normally contribute less than 20% of the total airway resistance. Therefore, changes in them are difficult to detect, and they constitute a "silent zone." However, it is likely that some of the earliest changes in COPD occur in these small airways, and therefore, maximum flow rate late in a forced expiration is often taken to reflect peripheral airway resistance.

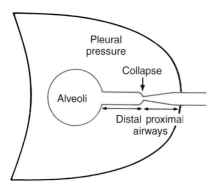

Figure 1.7. Dynamic compression of the airways. When this occurs during a forced expiration, only the resistance of the airways distal to the point of collapse (upstream segment) determines the flow rate. In the last stages of a forced vital capacity test, only the peripheral small airways are distal to the collapsed point and therefore determine the flow.

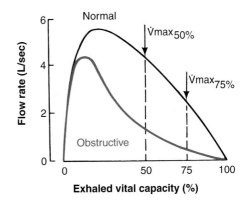

Figure 1.8. Example of an expiratory flow–volume curve in COPD. Note the scooped-out appearance. The *arrows* show the maximum expiratory flow after 50% and 75% of the vital capacity have been exhaled.

Maximum Flows from the Flow–Volume Curve

Maximum flow ($\dot{V}$ max) is frequently measured after 50% ($\dot{V}$ max$_{50\%}$) or 75% ($\dot{V}$ max$_{75\%}$) of the vital capacity has been exhaled. **Figure 1.8** shows the abnormal flow pattern typically seen in tests of patients with COPD. The later in expiration that the flow is measured, the more the measurement reflects the resistance of the very small airways. Some studies have shown abnormalities in the $\dot{V}$ max$_{75\%}$ when other indices of a forced expiration, such as the FEV$_1$ or FEF$_{25-75\%}$, were normal.

Peak Expiratory Flow Rate

Peak expiratory flow rate is the maximum flow rate during a forced expiration starting from total lung capacity. It can be conveniently estimated with an inexpensive, portable peak flow meter. The measurement is not precise, and it depends on the patient's effort. Nevertheless, it is a valuable tool for following disease, especially asthma, and the patient can easily make repeated measurements in the home or workplace and keep a log to show to the physician.

Inspiratory Flow–Volume Curve

The flow–volume curve is also often measured during inspiration. This curve is not affected by the dynamic compression of the airways because the pressures during inspiration always expand the bronchi (Figure 1.6). However, the curve is useful in detecting upper airway obstruction, which flattens the curve because maximal flow is limited **(Figure 1.9)**. Causes include glottic and tracheal stenosis and tracheal narrowing as a result of a compressing neoplasm. In fixed (nonvariable) obstruction, the expiratory flow–volume curve is also flattened.

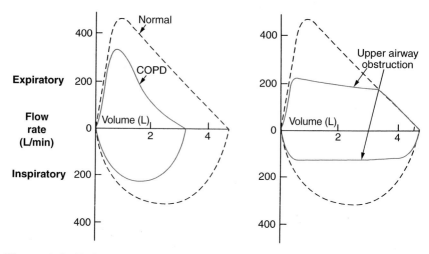

Figure 1.9. Expiratory and inspiratory flow–volume curves. In normal subjects and patients with COPD, inspiratory flow rates are normal (or nearly so). In fixed upper airway obstruction, both inspiratory and expiratory flow rates are reduced.

TESTS OF UNEVEN VENTILATION

Single-Breath Nitrogen Test

The tests described so far measure ventilatory capacity. The single-breath nitrogen test measures inequality of ventilation. This topic is somewhat different but is conveniently described here.

Suppose a patient takes a vital capacity inspiration of oxygen, that is, to total lung capacity, and then exhales slowly as far as he can, that is, to residual volume. If we measure the nitrogen concentration at the mouthpiece with a rapid nitrogen analyzer, we record a pattern as shown in **Figure 1.10**. Four phases can be recognized. In the first, which is very short, pure oxygen is exhaled from the upper airways, and the nitrogen concentration is zero. In the second phase, the nitrogen concentration rises rapidly as the anatomic dead space is washed out by alveolar gas. This phase is also short.

The third phase consists of alveolar gas, and the tracing is nearly flat with a small upward slope in normal subjects. This portion is often known as the alveolar plateau. In patients with uneven ventilation, the third phase is steeper, and the slope is a measure of the inequality of ventilation. It is expressed as the percentage increase in nitrogen concentration per liter of expired volume. In carrying out this test, the expiratory flow rate should be no more than 0.5 L/sec in order to reduce the variability of the results.

The reason for the rise in nitrogen concentration in phase 4 is that some regions of the lung are poorly ventilated and therefore receive relatively little of the breath of oxygen. These areas therefore have a relatively high

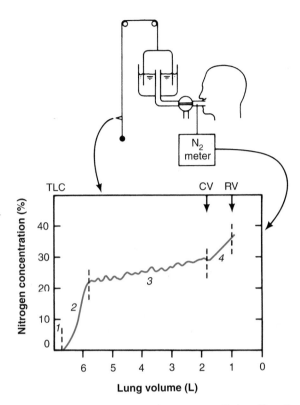

Figure 1.10. Single-breath nitrogen test of uneven ventilation. Note the four phases of the expired tracing. *TLC*, total lung capacity; *CV*, closing volume; *RV*, residual volume.

concentration of nitrogen because there is less oxygen to dilute this gas. Also, these poorly ventilated regions tend to empty last.

Three possible mechanisms of uneven ventilation are shown in **Figure 1.11**. In Figure 1.11A, the region is poorly ventilated because of partial obstruction of its airway, and because of this high resistance, the region empties late. In fact, the rate of emptying of such a region is determined by its time constant, which is given by the product of its airway resistance (R) and compliance (C). The larger the time constant (RC), the longer it takes to empty. This mechanism is known as *parallel* inequality of ventilation.

Figure 1.11B shows the mechanism known as *series* inequality. Here, there is a dilation of peripheral airspaces, which causes differences of ventilation *along* the air passages of a lung unit. In this context, we should recall that inspired gas reaches the terminal bronchioles by convective flow, that is, like water running through a hose, but its subsequent movement to the alveoli is chiefly accomplished by diffusion within the airways. Normally, the distances are so short that nearly complete equilibration of gas concentrations is established quickly. However, if the small airways enlarge, as occurs, for example, in centriacinar emphysema (see Figure 4.4), the concentration of inspired gas in the most distal airways may remain low. Again, these poorly ventilated regions empty last.

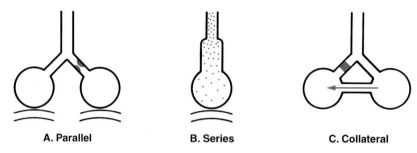

A. Parallel   **B. Series**   **C. Collateral**

Figure 1.11. Three mechanisms of uneven ventilation. In parallel inequality **(A)**, flow to regions with long time constants is reduced. In series inequality **(B)**, dilation of a small airway may result in incomplete diffusion along a terminal lung unit. Collateral ventilation **(C)** may also cause series inequality.

Figure 1.11C shows another form of series inequality that occurs when some lung units receive their inspired gas from neighboring units rather than from the large airways. This is known as collateral ventilation and appears to be an important process in COPD and asthma.

Uneven Ventilation

- Occurs in many patients with lung disease
- Is an important factor contributing to impaired gas exchange
- Is conveniently measured with the single-breath N_2 test

There is still uncertainty about the relative importance of parallel and series inequality. It is likely that both operate to a small extent in people with normal ventilation and to a much greater degree in patients with obstructive pulmonary disease. Whatever the mechanism, the single-breath nitrogen test is a simple, rapid, and reliable way of measuring the degree of uneven ventilation in the lung. This is increased in most obstructive and many restrictive types of lung disease (see Chapters 4 and 5).

Closing Volume

Toward the end of the vital capacity expiration shown in Figure 1.10, the nitrogen concentration rises abruptly, signaling the onset of airway closure, or phase 4. The lung volume at which phase 4 begins is called the *closing volume*, and the closing volume plus the residual volume is known as the *closing capacity*. In practice, the onset of phase 4 is obtained by drawing a straight line through the alveolar plateau (phase 3) and noting the last point of departure of the nitrogen tracing from this line.

Unfortunately, the junction between phases 3 and 4 is seldom as clear-cut as in Figure 1.10, and there is considerable variation of this volume when the test is repeated by a patient. The test is most useful in the presence of small amounts of disease because severe disease distorts the tracing so much that the closing volume cannot be identified.

The mechanism of the onset of phase 4 is still uncertain but is believed to be closure of small airways in the lowest part of the lung. At residual volume just before the single breath of oxygen is inhaled, the nitrogen concentration is virtually uniform throughout the lung, but the basal alveoli are much smaller than the apical alveoli in the upright subject because of distortion of the lung by its weight. Indeed, the lowest portions are compressed so much that the small airways in the region of the respiratory bronchioles are closed. However, at the end of a vital capacity inspiration, all the alveoli are approximately the same size. Thus, the nitrogen at the base is diluted much more than that at the apex by the breath of oxygen.

During the subsequent expiration, the upper and lower zones empty together and the expired nitrogen concentration is nearly constant (Figure 1.10). As soon as dependent airways begin to close, however, the higher nitrogen concentration in the upper zones preferentially affects the expired concentration, causing an abrupt rise. Moreover, as airway closure proceeds up the lung, the expired nitrogen progressively increases.

Some studies show that in some subjects, the closing volume is the same in the weightlessness of space as in normal gravity. This finding suggests that compression of a dependent lung is not always the mechanism.

The volume at which airways close is age dependent, being as low as 10% of the vital capacity in young normal subjects but increasing to 40% (i.e., approximately the FRC) at about the age of 65 years. There is some evidence that the test is sensitive to small amounts of disease. For example, apparently healthy cigarette smokers sometimes have increased closing volumes when their ventilatory capacity is normal.

Other Tests of Uneven Ventilation

Uneven ventilation can also be measured by a multibreath nitrogen washout during oxygen breathing. Topographic inequality of ventilation can be determined using radioactive xenon. This chapter is confined to single-breath tests; other measurements are referred to in Chapter 3.

Tests of Early Airway Disease

There has been interest in the possible use of some tests described in this chapter to identify patients with early airway disease. Once a patient develops the full picture of COPD, considerable, irreversible parenchymal damage has already been done. The hope is that by identifying disease at an early stage, its progression can be slowed, for example, by the patient stopping cigarette smoking.

Among the tests that have been examined in this context are the FEV_1, $FEF_{25-75\%}$, $\dot{V}max_{50\%}$ and $\dot{V}max_{75\%}$, and the closing volume. Assessment of these tests is difficult because it depends on prospective studies and large control groups. It is now clear that the original test of FEV_1 remains one of the most reliable and valuable tests. While more sophisticated tests should be investigated, measuring the FEV_1 and FVC remains mandatory.

KEY CONCEPTS

1. The 1-second forced expiratory volume and the forced vital capacity are easy tests to do, require little equipment, and are often very informative.

2. Dynamic compression of the airways is common in COPD and is a major cause of disability.

3. The small airways (less than 2 mm in diameter) are often the site of early airway disease, but the changes are difficult to detect.

4. Uneven ventilation is common in airway diseases and can be measured with a single-breath N_2 test.

5. The closing volume is often increased in mild airway disease, and it also increases with age.

CLINICAL VIGNETTE

A 30-year-old man complains of increasing dyspnea over a 2-week period. He states that he is no longer able to maintain the same pace on his daily runs and adds that he feels more out of breath when he lies flat on his back at night. He is a non-smoker and works as a software designer. He also notes that he has been sweating more than usual when he sleeps at night and has lost about 3 kg of weight despite not changing his diet or physical activity. On physical exam, he has no wheezing on auscultation. When he is placed in the supine position for the cardiac exam, he is noted to have increased dyspnea, which resolves when he reassumes the upright position. Spirometry shows the following:

Parameter	Predicted Value	Prebron-chodilator	% Predicted	Postbron-chodilator	% Predicted
FEV_1 (L)	4.5	2.9	64	3.1	69
FVC (L)	5.2	4.2	81	4.2	81
FEV_1/FVC	0.87	0.69	—	0.74	—

CLINICAL VIGNETTE (*Continued*)

Flow–Volume Curve

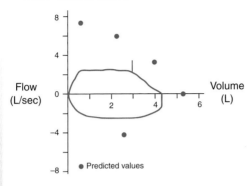

Questions

- How would you interpret the numerical values from his spirometry?
- Are there any changes in his pulmonary function with bronchodilator administration?
- What information does the flow–volume curve add about the cause of his problem?

QUESTIONS

For each question, choose the best answer.

1. The inspiratory flow–volume curve is most valuable for:
   A. Detecting fixed upper airway obstruction.
   B. Measuring the response to bronchodilator drugs.
   C. Differentiating between chronic bronchitis and emphysema.
   D. Detecting resistance in small peripheral airways.
   E. Detecting fatigue of the diaphragm.

2. Concerning the single-breath nitrogen test:
   A. It is usually normal in mild COPD.
   B. The slope of phase 3 is increased in chronic bronchitis.
   C. In phase 3, well-ventilated units empty last.
   D. In normal subjects, the last expired gas comes from the base of the lung.
   E. The expiratory flow rate should be as fast as possible.

3. The closing volume as measured from the single-breath N_2 test:
A. Decreases with age.
B. Is highly reproducible.
C. Is affected by the small, peripheral airways.
D. Is most informative in patients with severe lung disease.
E. Is normal in mild COPD.

4. A 72-year-old woman who is a heavy smoker complains of worsening dyspnea and a productive cough over a 9-month period. Spirometry shows an FEV_1 1.1 liters, an FVC 2.8 liters, and an FEV_1/FVC ratio of 0.39. Which of the following mechanisms best accounts for the results of these tests?
A. Decreased lung compliance
B. Dynamic compression of the airways
C. Increased radial traction on the airways
D. Increased thickness of the blood–gas barrier
E. Weakness of the diaphragm

5. A 61-year-old man with a 30-pack-year history of smoking complains of worsening dyspnea and a dry cough over a 6-month period. Spirometry shows an FEV_1 of 1.9 liters, an FVC of 2.2 liters, and an FEV_1/FVC ratio of 0.86. Which of the following diseases is consistent with this presentation?
A. Asthma
B. Chronic bronchitis
C. Chronic obstructive pulmonary disease
D. Pulmonary fibrosis
E. Pulmonary hypertension

6. A 41-year-old woman performs spirometry because she complains of dyspnea. She did not give a full effort on the first test and was asked by the laboratory technologist to repeat the test a second time. Which of the following changes in her spirometry would you expect to see if she makes a better effort on the second trial?
A. Decreased vital capacity
B. Flattening of the expiratory limb of the flow–volume loop
C. Flattening on the inspiratory limb of the flow–volume loop
D. Increased expiratory flow at end exhalation
E. Increased peak expiratory flow rate

7. A 57-year-old man undergoes spirometry because of chronic dyspnea on exertion. The flow–volume loop is depicted in the figure below. The blue dots show the predicted values. Which of the following factors could account for the shape of the flow–volume curve?

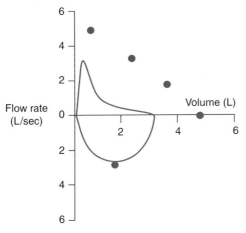

A. Fibrosis of the lung parenchyma
B. Increased radial traction on the airways
C. Increased elastic recoil
D. Increased airway secretions
E. Increased number of pulmonary capillaries

GAS EXCHANGE

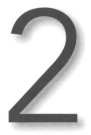

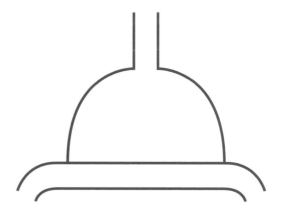

- **Blood Gases**
  Arterial P_{O_2}
    Measurement
    Normal Values
    Causes of Hypoxemia
    Intermittent Hypoxemia
  Arterial P_{CO_2}
    Measurement
    Normal Values
    Causes of Increased
      Arterial P_{CO_2}
  Arterial pH
    Measurement
    Acidosis
    Alkalosis

- **Diffusing Capacity**
  Measurement of Diffusing
    Capacity
  Causes of Reduced Diffusing
    Capacity
  Interpretation of Diffusing
    Capacity

Chapter 1 dealt with the simplest test of lung function: the forced expiration. In addition, we looked briefly at the single-breath test of uneven ventilation. In this chapter, we turn to the most important measurement in the management of respiratory failure: arterial blood gases. Another test of gas exchange, the diffusing capacity, is also discussed.

BLOOD GASES

Arterial P_{O_2}

Measurement

It is often essential to know the partial pressure of oxygen in the arterial blood of acutely ill patients. With modern blood gas electrodes, the measurement of arterial P_{O_2} is relatively simple, and the test is mandatory in the management of patients with respiratory failure.

Arterial blood is usually taken by puncturing the radial artery or from an indwelling radial artery catheter. The P_{O_2} is measured by the polarographic principle, that is, the test measures the current that flows when a small voltage is applied to electrodes.

Normal Values

The normal value for P_{O_2} in young adults at or near sea level averages approximately 90 to 95 mm Hg, with a range of approximately 85 to 100 mm Hg. The normal value decreases steadily with age, and the average is approximately 85 mm Hg at age 60 years. The cause of the fall in P_{O_2} with age is probably increasing ventilation–perfusion inequality (see the section later in this chapter).

Whenever we report an arterial P_{O_2} test, we should have the oxygen dissociation curve at the back of our minds. **Figure 2.1** reminds us of two anchor points on the normal curve. One is arterial blood (P_{O_2}, 100; O_2 saturation,

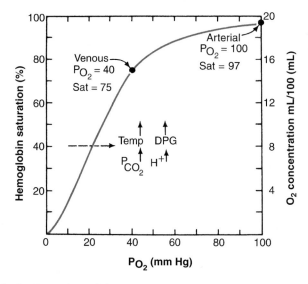

Figure 2.1. Anchor points of the oxygen dissociation curve. The curve is shifted to the right by an increase in temperature, P_{CO_2}, H^+, and 2,3-DPG. The oxygen concentration scale is based on a hemoglobin concentration of 14.5 g/100 mL.

97%) and the other is mixed venous blood (P_{O_2}, 40; O_2 saturation, 75%). Also we should recall that above 60 mm Hg, the O_2 saturation exceeds 90% and the curve is fairly flat. The curve is shifted to the right by an increase in temperature, P_{CO_2}, and H^+ concentration (these all occur in exercising muscle when enhanced unloading of O_2 is advantageous). The curve is also shifted to the right by an increase in 2,3-diphosphoglycerate (DPG) inside the red cells. 2,3-DPG is depleted in stored blood but is increased in prolonged hypoxia.

Causes of Hypoxemia

There are four primary causes of a reduced P_{O_2} in arterial blood:

1. Hypoventilation
2. Diffusion impairment
3. Shunt
4. Ventilation–perfusion inequality

A fifth cause, reduction of inspired P_{O_2}, is seen only in special circumstances such as at high altitude or when breathing a gas mixture of low oxygen concentration.

Hypoventilation

This means that the volume of fresh gas going to the alveoli per unit time (alveolar ventilation) is reduced. If the resting oxygen consumption is not correspondingly reduced, hypoxemia inevitably results. Hypoventilation is commonly caused by diseases outside the lungs; indeed, very often, the lungs are normal.

Two cardinal physiologic features of hypoventilation should be emphasized. First, it *always* causes a rise in P_{CO_2}, and this is a valuable diagnostic feature. The relationship between the arterial P_{CO_2} and the level of alveolar ventilation in the normal lung is a simple one and is given by the *alveolar ventilation equation*:

$$P_{CO_2} = \frac{\dot{V}_{CO_2}}{\dot{V}_A} \cdot K, \qquad \text{(Eq. 2.1)}$$

where $\dot{V}_{CO_2}$ is the CO_2 output, $\dot{V}_A$ is the alveolar ventilation, and K is a constant (see Appendix A for a list of symbols). This means that if the alveolar ventilation is halved, the P_{CO_2} is doubled. If the patient does not have a raised arterial P_{CO_2}, he or she is not hypoventilating!

Second, the hypoxemia can be abolished easily by increasing the inspired P_{O_2} by delivering oxygen via a face mask. This can be seen from the *alveolar gas equation*:

$$P_{A_{O_2}} = P_{I_{O_2}} - \frac{P_{A_{CO_2}}}{R} + F, \qquad \text{(Eq. 2.2)}$$

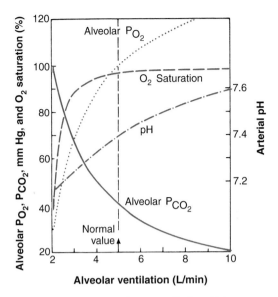

Figure 2.2. Gas exchange during hypoventilation. Values are approximate.

where F is a small correction factor that can be ignored. We will also assume that the alveolar and arterial P_{CO_2} values are the same. This equation states that if the arterial P_{CO_2} ($P_{A_{CO_2}}$) and respiratory exchange ratio (R) remain constant (they will, if the alveolar ventilation and metabolic rate remain unaltered), every mm Hg rise in inspired P_{O_2} ($P_{I_{O_2}}$) produces a corresponding rise in the alveolar P_{O_2} ($P_{A_{O_2}}$). Because it is easily possible to increase the inspired P_{O_2} by several hundred mm Hg, the hypoxemia of pure hypoventilation can readily be abolished.

It is also important to appreciate that the arterial P_{O_2} cannot fall to very low levels from pure hypoventilation. Referring to Equation 2.2 again, we can see that if R = 1, the alveolar P_{O_2} falls 1 mm Hg for every 1 mm Hg rise in P_{CO_2}. This means that severe hypoventilation sufficient to double the P_{CO_2} from 40 to 80 mm Hg only decreases the alveolar P_{O_2} from, say, 100 to 60 mm Hg. If R = 0.8, the fall is somewhat greater, say, to 50 mm Hg. Also, the arterial P_{O_2} is usually a few mm Hg lower than the alveolar value. Even so, the arterial O_2 saturation will be near 80% **(Figure 2.2)**. However, this is a severe degree of CO_2 retention that may result in substantial respiratory acidosis, a pH of around 7.2, and a very sick patient! Thus, hypoxemia is not the dominant feature of hypoventilation.

The causes of hypoventilation are shown in **Figure 2.3** and listed in **Table 2.1**. In addition, hypoventilation is seen in some extremely obese patients who have somnolence, polycythemia, and excessive appetite. This has been dubbed the "pickwickian syndrome" after the fat boy, Joe, in Charles Dickens's *Pickwick Papers*. The cause of the hypoventilation is uncertain, but

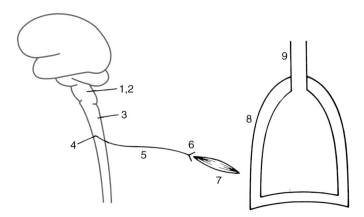

Figure 2.3. **Causes of hypoventilation.** (See Table 2.1 for details.)

the increased work of breathing associated with obesity is probably a factor, although some patients appear to have an abnormality of the central nervous system. There is also a rare condition of idiopathic hypoventilation known as Ondine's curse.

Diffusion Impairment

This means that equilibration does not occur between the P_{O_2} in the pulmonary capillary blood and alveolar gas. **Figure 2.4** reminds us of the time course for P_{O_2} along a pulmonary capillary. Under normal resting conditions, the capillary blood P_{O_2} almost reaches that of alveolar gas after about 1/3 of the total contact time of 3/4 second available in the capillary. Thus, there is plenty of time in reserve. Even with severe exercise, when the contact time may perhaps be reduced to as little as 1/4 second, equilibration almost always occurs.

Table 2.1	Some Causes of Hypoventilation (see Figure 2.3)

1. Depression of the respiratory center by drugs (e.g., barbiturates and morphine derivatives)
2. Diseases of the medulla (e.g., encephalitis, hemorrhage, neoplasms [rare])
3. Abnormalities of the spinal cord (e.g., following high cervical spinal cord injury)
4. Anterior horn cell disease (e.g., poliomyelitis)
5. Diseases of the nerves to the respiratory muscles (e.g., in the Guillain-Barré syndrome or diphtheria)
6. Diseases of the myoneural junction (e.g., myasthenia gravis, anticholinesterase poisoning)
7. Diseases of the respiratory muscles (e.g., Duchenne muscular dystrophy)
8. Thoracic cage abnormalities (e.g., crushed chest)
9. Upper airway obstruction (e.g., tracheal compression by enlarged lymph nodes)

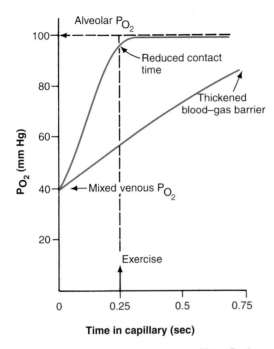

Figure 2.4. Changes in P$_{O_2}$ along the pulmonary capillary. During exercise, the time available for O$_2$ diffusion across the blood–gas barrier is reduced. A thickened alveolar wall slows the rate of diffusion.

However, in some diseases, the blood–gas barrier is thickened and diffusion is so slowed that equilibration may be incomplete. **Figure 2.5** shows a histologic section of lung from a patient with interstitial fibrosis. Note that the normally delicate alveolar walls are grossly widened. In such a lung, we expect a slower time course, as shown in Figure 2.4. Any hypoxemia that occurred at rest would be exaggerated on exercise because of the reduced contact time between blood and gas.

Diseases in which diffusion impairment may contribute to the hypoxemia, especially on exercise, include asbestosis, sarcoidosis, diffuse interstitial fibrosis including idiopathic pulmonary fibrosis (cryptogenic fibrosing alveolitis) and interstitial pneumonia, connective tissue diseases affecting the lung including scleroderma, rheumatoid lung, lupus erythematosus, granulomatosis with polyangiitis (also known as Wegener's granulomatosis), Goodpasture's syndrome, and adenocarcinoma in situ. In all these conditions, the diffusion path from alveolar gas to red blood cell may be increased, at least in some regions of the lung, and the time course for oxygenation may be affected, as shown in Figure 2.4.

However, the importance of diffusion impairment to the arterial hypoxemia in these patients is less than it was once thought to be. As has been emphasized, the normal lung has lots of diffusion time in reserve. In addition,

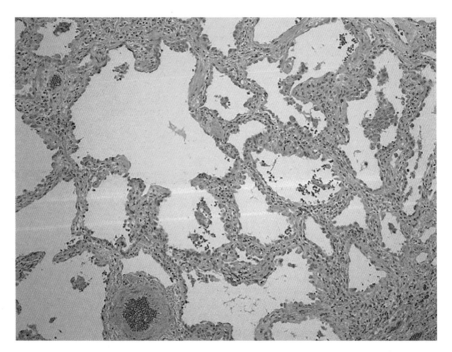

Figure 2.5. Section of lung from a patient with idiopathic pulmonary fibrosis. Note the extreme thickening of the alveolar walls, which constitutes a barrier to diffusion (compare with Figures 5.1, 5.3, and 10.5). (Image courtesy of Corinne Fligner, MD.)

if we look at Figure 2.5, it is impossible to believe that the normal relationships between ventilation and blood flow can be preserved in a lung with such an abnormal architecture. We will see shortly that ventilation–perfusion inequality is a powerful cause of hypoxemia, which is undoubtedly operating in these patients. Thus, how much additional hypoxemia should be attributed to diffusion impairment is difficult to know. It is clear that at least some of the hypoxemia on exercise is caused by this mechanism (see Figure 5.6).

Hypoxemia could also result from an extreme reduction in contact time. Suppose that so much blood flow is diverted away from other regions of the lung (e.g., by a large pulmonary embolus) that the time for oxygenation within the capillary is reduced to one-tenth normal. Figure 2.4 shows that hypoxemia would then be inevitable.

Hypoxemia caused by diffusion impairment can be corrected readily by administering 100% oxygen to the patient. The resultant large increase in alveolar P_{O_2} of several hundred mm Hg can easily overcome the increased diffusion resistance of the thickened blood–gas barrier. Carbon dioxide elimination is generally unaffected by diffusion abnormalities. Most patients with the diseases listed earlier do not have carbon dioxide retention. Indeed, typically, the arterial P_{CO_2} is slightly lower than normal because ventilation is overstimulated, either by the hypoxemia or by intrapulmonary receptors.

Shunt

A shunt allows some blood to reach the arterial system without passing through ventilated regions of the lung. Intrapulmonary shunts can be caused by arterial–venous malformations that often have a genetic basis. In addition, an unventilated but perfused area of lung, for example, a consolidated pneumonic lobule, constitutes a shunt. It might be argued that the latter example is simply one extreme of the spectrum of ventilation–perfusion ratios and that it is therefore more reasonable to classify hypoxemia caused by this under the heading of ventilation–perfusion inequality. However, shunt causes such a characteristic pattern of gas exchange during 100% oxygen breathing that it is convenient to include unventilated alveoli under this heading. Very large shunts are often seen in the acute respiratory distress syndrome (see Chapter 8). Many shunts are extrapulmonary, including those that occur in congenital heart disease through atrial or ventricular septal defects or a patent foramen ovale. In such patients, there must be a rise in right heart pressure to cause a shunt from right to left.

If a patient with a shunt is given pure oxygen to breathe, the arterial P_{O_2} fails to rise to the level seen in normal subjects. **Figure 2.6** shows that although the end-capillary P_{O_2} may be as high as that in alveolar gas, the O_2

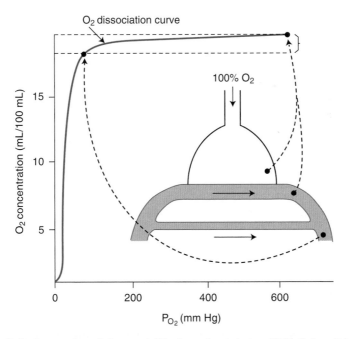

Figure 2.6. Depression of the arterial P_{O_2} by a shunt during 100% O_2 breathing. The addition of a small amount of shunted blood with its low O_2 concentration greatly reduces the O_2 of arterial blood. This is because the O_2 dissociation curve is so flat when the P_{O_2} is high.

concentration of the shunted blood is as low as in venous blood if the shunt is mixed venous blood. When a small amount of shunted blood is added to arterial blood, the O_2 concentration is depressed. This causes a large fall in arterial P_{O_2} because the O_2 dissociation curve is so flat in its upper range. As a result, it is possible to detect small shunts by measuring the arterial P_{O_2} during 100% O_2 breathing.

Only shunts behave in this way and this is a point of practical importance. In the other three causes of hypoxemia (hypoventilation, diffusion impairment, and ventilation–perfusion inequality), the arterial P_{O_2} nearly reaches the normal level seen in healthy subjects during 100% O_2 breathing. This may take a long time in some patients who have poorly ventilated alveoli because the nitrogen takes so long to wash out completely that the P_{O_2} is slow to reach its final level. This is probably the reason why the arterial P_{O_2} of patients with chronic obstructive pulmonary disease (COPD) may only rise to 400 to 500 mm Hg after 15 minutes of 100% O_2 breathing.

If the shunt is caused by mixed venous blood, its magnitude during O_2 breathing can be determined from the *shunt equation*:

$$\frac{\dot{Q}_S}{\dot{Q}_T} = \frac{C_{C'} - C_a}{C_{C'} - C_{\bar{V}}}, \qquad\qquad \text{(Eq. 2.3)}$$

where $\dot{Q}_S$ and $\dot{Q}_T$ refer to the shunt and total blood flows, and $C_{c'}$, C_a, and $C_{\bar{v}}$ refer to the O_2 concentrations of end-capillary, arterial, and mixed venous blood. The O_2 concentration of the end-capillary blood is calculated from the alveolar P_{O_2}, assuming complete equilibration between the alveolar gas and the blood. Mixed venous blood is sampled with a catheter in the pulmonary artery. The denominator in Equation 2.3 can also be estimated from the measured oxygen uptake and cardiac output.

Shunt does not usually result in a raised arterial P_{CO_2}. The tendency for this to rise is generally countered by the chemoreceptors, which increase ventilation if the P_{CO_2} increases. Indeed, often the arterial P_{CO_2} is lower than normal because of the additional hypoxemic stimulus to ventilation.

Ventilation–Perfusion Inequality
In this condition, ventilation and blood flow are mismatched in various regions of the lung, with the result that all gas transfer becomes inefficient. This mechanism of hypoxemia is extremely common; it is responsible for most, if not all, of the hypoxemia of COPD, interstitial lung disease, and vascular disorders such as pulmonary embolism. It is often identified by excluding the other three causes of hypoxemia: hypoventilation, diffusion impairment, and shunt.

All lungs have some ventilation–perfusion inequality. In the normal upright lung, this takes the form of a regional pattern, with the ventilation–perfusion ratio decreasing from apex to base. But if pulmonary disease occurs and progresses, we see a disorganization of this pattern until eventually the normal relationships between ventilation and blood flow are destroyed at the alveolar level. (For a discussion of the physiology of how ventilation–perfusion inequality causes hypoxemia, see the companion volume, *West's Respiratory Physiology: The Essentials*. 10th ed. pp. 70–82.)

Several factors can exaggerate the hypoxemia of ventilation–perfusion inequality. One is concomitant hypoventilation, which may occur, for example, if a patient with severe COPD is overly sedated. Another factor that is frequently overlooked is a reduction in cardiac output. This causes a fall of P_{O_2} in mixed venous blood, which results in a fall of arterial P_{O_2} for the same degree of ventilation–perfusion inequality. This situation may be seen in patients who develop a myocardial infarct with mild pulmonary edema.

How can we assess the severity of ventilation–perfusion inequality from the arterial blood gases? First, the *arterial* P_{O_2} is a useful guide. A patient with an arterial P_{O_2} of 40 mm Hg is likely to have more ventilation–perfusion inequality than a patient with an arterial P_{O_2} of 70 mm Hg. However, we can be misled. For example, suppose that the first patient had reduced the ventilation, with the result that the alveolar P_{O_2} had fallen by 30 mm Hg, thus pulling down the arterial P_{O_2}. Under these conditions, the arterial P_{O_2} by itself would be deceptive. For this reason, we often calculate the *alveolar–arterial difference* for P_{O_2}.

What value should we use for alveolar P_{O_2}? **Figure 2.7** reminds us that in a lung with ventilation–perfusion ($\dot{V}_A/\dot{Q}$) inequality, there may be a wide spectrum of values for alveolar P_{O_2} ranging from inspired gas to mixed venous blood. A solution is to calculate an "ideal alveolar P_{O_2}." This is the value that the lung *would* have if there were no ventilation–perfusion inequality and

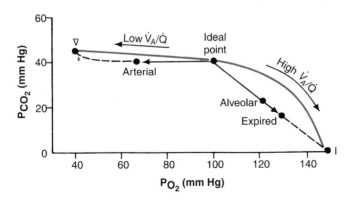

Figure 2.7. O_2– CO_2 diagram showing the mixed venous ($\bar{v}$), inspired (I), arterial, ideal, alveolar, and expired points. The curved line indicates the P_{O_2} and P_{CO_2} of all lung units having different ventilation–perfusion ($\dot{V}_A/\dot{Q}$) ratios. (For additional information on this difficult topic, see *West's Respiratory Physiology: The Essentials*. 10th ed. pp. 70–78.)

if the respiratory exchange ratio remained the same. It is found from the *alveolar gas equation*:

$$P_{A_{O_2}} = P_{I_{O_2}} - \frac{P_{A_{CO_2}}}{R} + F, \qquad (Eq.\ 2.4)$$

using the respiratory exchange ratio R of the whole lung and assuming that arterial and alveolar P_{CO_2} are the same (usually they nearly are). Thus, the alveolar–arterial difference for P_{O_2} makes an allowance for the effect of under-ventilation or overventilation on the arterial P_{O_2} and is a purer measure of ventilation–perfusion inequality. Other indices include the physiologic dead space and physiologic shunt. (See *West's Respiratory Physiology: The Essentials.* 10th ed. pp. 187–189 for further details.)

It is possible to obtain more information about the distribution of ventilation–perfusion ratios in the lung with a technique based on the elimination of injected foreign gases in solution. The details will not be given here, but it is thus possible to derive a virtually continuous distribution of ventilation–perfusion ratios that is consistent with the measured pattern of the elimination of the six gases. **Figure 2.8** shows a typical pattern found in young normal volunteers. It can be seen that almost all the ventilation and blood flow go to lung units with ventilation–perfusion ratios near the normal value of 1. As we shall see in Chapter 4, this pattern is greatly disturbed by lung disease.

Mixed Causes of Hypoxemia

These frequently occur. For example, a patient who is being mechanically ventilated because of acute respiratory failure after an automobile collision

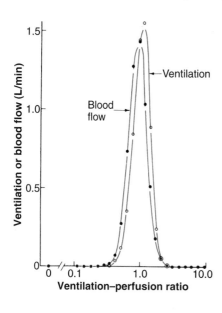

Figure 2.8. Distribution of ventilation–perfusion ratios in a young normal subject as obtained by the multiple inert gas elimination technique. Note that most of the ventilation and blood flow go to lung units with ventilation–perfusion ratios near 1. (From Wagner PD, Laravuso RB, Uhl RR, West JB. Continuous distributions of ventilation–perfusion ratios in normal subjects breathing air and 100% O_2. *J Clin Invest* 1974;54:54–68.)

may have a large shunt through the unventilated lung in addition to severe ventilation–perfusion inequality (see Figure 8.3). Again, a patient with interstitial lung disease may have some diffusion impairment, but this is certainly accompanied by ventilation–perfusion inequality and possibly by shunt as well (see Figures 5.7 and 5.8). In our present state of knowledge, it is often impossible to define accurately the mechanism of hypoxemia, especially in the severely ill patient.

Intermittent Hypoxemia

While hypoxemia may last for days to weeks in patients with pneumonia or the acute respiratory distress syndrome or be a permanent problem in some patients with COPD or pulmonary fibrosis, it can also occur in recurrent brief episodes of less than a minute in duration. This intermittent form of hypoxemia is seen most commonly in patients with sleep disordered breathing, of which there are two primary variants, *central sleep apnea*, where there are no respiratory efforts, and *obstructive sleep apnea*, where, despite activity of the respiratory muscles, there is no airflow.

Central sleep apnea often occurs in patients with severe heart failure and various forms of central nervous system injury and can also be seen in normal people at high altitude. In one particular form of central sleep apnea, referred to as Cheyne-Stokes breathing, there are alternating periods of breathing, in which the tidal volume waxes and wanes in a crescendo–decrescendo pattern, and periods of apnea. This is thought to occur as a result of instability in the feedback control system that regulates breathing patterns during sleep.

Obstructive sleep apnea is the more common pattern of sleep disordered breathing. The first reports were in obese patients, but it is now recognized that the condition is not confined to them. Airway obstruction can be caused by backward movement of the tongue, collapse of the pharyngeal walls, greatly enlarged tonsils or adenoids, and other anatomic causes of pharyngeal narrowing. With inspiration, the pressure within the airway falls, predisposing to airway collapse. Loud snoring often occurs, and the patient may wake violently after an apneic episode. Chronic sleep deprivation sometimes occurs, and the patient may have daytime somnolence, impaired cognitive function, chronic fatigue, morning headaches, and personality disturbances such as paranoia, hostility, and agitated depression. Untreated patients are at risk for cardiovascular complications such as systemic hypertension, coronary artery disease and stroke, possibly as a result of increased sympathetic nervous system activity during apneic episodes. Application of continuous positive airway pressure (CPAP) by means of a full face or nasal mask during sleep raises the pressure inside the airway, thus acting as a pneumatic splint. While this is generally seen as the most effective treatment, some patients are unable to tolerate it and surgical approaches may be necessary.

In addition to these pathological forms of intermittent hypoxemia, there has been recent interest in the concept of ischemic preconditioning whereby brief periods of hypoxemia are intentionally induced as a means of protecting against subsequent ischemic injury that might occur in a myocardial infarction or acute limb ischemia due to peripheral vascular disease.

Oxygen Delivery to Tissues

Although the P_{O_2} of arterial blood is of great importance, other factors enter into the delivery of oxygen to the tissues. For example, a reduced arterial P_{O_2} is clearly more detrimental in a patient with a hemoglobin of 5 g/100 mL than it is in a patient with a normal O_2 capacity. The delivery of oxygen to the tissues depends on the oxygen concentration of the blood, the cardiac output, and the distribution of blood flow to the periphery. These factors are discussed further in Chapter 9.

Arterial P_{CO_2}

Measurement

A P_{CO_2} electrode is essentially a glass pH electrode. This is surrounded by a bicarbonate buffer, which is separated from the blood by a thin membrane through which CO_2 diffuses. The CO_2 alters the pH of the buffer, and this is measured by the electrode, which reads out the P_{CO_2} directly.

Normal Values

The normal arterial P_{CO_2} is 37 to 43 mm Hg and is almost unaffected by age. It tends to fall in the late stages of heavy exercise and to rise slightly during sleep. Sometimes a blood sample obtained by arterial puncture shows a value in the mid-30s. This can be attributed to the acute hyperventilation caused by the procedure and can be recognized by the correspondingly increased pH.

Causes of Increased Arterial P_{CO_2}

There are two major causes of CO_2 retention: hypoventilation and ventilation–perfusion inequality.

Hypoventilation

This was dealt with in some detail earlier in the chapter, where we saw that hypoventilation must cause hypoxemia and CO_2 retention, the latter being more important (Figure 2.3). The *alveolar ventilation equation*

$$P_{A_{CO_2}} = \frac{\dot{V}_{CO_2}}{\dot{V}_A} \cdot K, \qquad \text{(Eq. 2.5)}$$

emphasizes the inverse relationship between the ventilation and the alveolar P_{CO_2}. In normal lungs, the arterial P_{CO_2} closely follows the alveolar value. Whereas the hypoxemia of hypoventilation can be relieved easily by increasing the inspired P_{O_2}, the CO_2 retention can only be treated by increasing the ventilation. This may require mechanical assistance as described in Chapter 10.

Ventilation–Perfusion Inequality

Although this condition was considered earlier, its relationship to CO_2 retention warrants a further brief discussion because of frequent confusion in this area. At one time, it was argued that ventilation–perfusion inequality does not interfere with CO_2 elimination because the overventilated regions make up for the underventilated areas. This is a fallacy, and it is important to realize that ventilation–perfusion inequality reduces the efficiency of transfer of all gases, including the anesthetic gases.

Why then do we frequently see patients with chronic pulmonary disease and undoubted ventilation–perfusion inequality who have a normal or even low arterial P_{CO_2}? **Figure 2.9** explains this. The normal relationships between ventilation and blood flow (A) are disturbed by disease, and hypoxemia and CO_2 retention develop (B). However, the chemoreceptors respond to the increased arterial P_{CO_2} and raise the ventilation to the alveoli. The result is that the arterial P_{CO_2} is returned to its normal level (C). However, although the arterial P_{O_2} is somewhat raised by the increased ventilation, it does not return all the way to normal. This can be explained by the shape of the O_2 dissociation curve and, in particular, the strongly depressive action on the arterial P_{O_2} of lung units with low ventilation–perfusion ratios. Whereas units with high ventilation–perfusion ratios are effective at eliminating CO_2, they have little advantage over normal units in taking up O_2. The end result is that the arterial P_{CO_2} is effectively lowered to the normal value, but there is relatively little rise in arterial P_{O_2}.

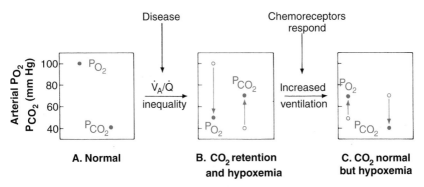

Figure 2.9. Arterial P_{O_2} and P_{CO_2} in different stages of ventilation–perfusion inequality. Initially, there must be both a fall in P_{O_2} and a rise in P_{CO_2}. However, when the ventilation to the alveoli is increased, the P_{CO_2} returns to normal but the P_{O_2} remains abnormally low.

Some patients do not make the transition from stage B to stage C or, having made it, revert to stage B and develop CO_2 retention. What is the reason for this? Generally, these patients have a high work of breathing, often because of a gross increase in airway resistance. Apparently, they elect to raise their P_{CO_2} rather than to expend the extra energy to increase ventilation. It is of interest that if normal subjects are made to breathe through a narrow tube, thus increasing their work of breathing, their alveolar P_{CO_2} often rises.

We do not fully understand why some patients with ventilation–perfusion inequality increase their ventilation and some do not. As we shall see in Chapter 5, many patients with emphysema hold their P_{CO_2} at the normal level even when their disease is far advanced. Patients with asthma generally do the same. This can involve a large increase in ventilation to their alveoli. However, other patients, for example, those with severe chronic bronchitis, typically allow their P_{CO_2} to rise much earlier in the course of the disease. It is possible that there is some difference in the central neurogenic control of ventilation in these two groups of patients.

Arterial pH

Measurement
Arterial pH is usually measured with a glass electrode concurrently with the arterial P_{O_2} and P_{CO_2}. It is related to the P_{CO_2} and bicarbonate concentration through the Henderson-Hasselbalch equation:

$$pH = pK + \log \frac{\left(HCO_3^-\right)}{0.03\,P_{CO_2}}, \qquad \text{(Eq. 2.6)}$$

where pK = 6.1, (HCO_3^-) is the plasma bicarbonate concentration in millimoles per liter, and the P_{CO_2} is in mm Hg.

Acidosis
Acidosis is a decrease in arterial pH or a process that tends to do this. Sometimes the term *acidemia* is used to refer to the actual fall in pH in the blood. Acidosis can be caused by respiratory or metabolic abnormalities or by both.

Respiratory Acidosis
This is caused by CO_2 retention, which increases the denominator in the Henderson-Hasselbalch equation and so depresses the pH. Both mechanisms of CO_2 retention (hypoventilation and ventilation–perfusion ratio inequality) can cause respiratory acidosis.

It is important to distinguish between acute and chronic CO_2 retention. A patient with hypoventilation after an overdose of opiates is likely to develop acute respiratory acidosis. There is little change in the bicarbonate concentration (the numerator in the Henderson-Hasselbalch equation), and the pH therefore falls rapidly as the P_{CO_2} rises. The base excess is normal in such cases. Typically, a doubling of the P_{CO_2} from 40 to 80 mm Hg in such a patient reduces the pH from 7.4 to approximately 7.2.

By contrast, a patient who develops chronic CO_2 retention over a period of many weeks as a result of increasing ventilation–perfusion inequality caused by chronic pulmonary disease typically has a smaller fall in pH. This is because the kidneys retain bicarbonate in response to the increased P_{CO_2} in the renal tubular cells, thus increasing the numerator in the Henderson-Hasselbalch equation (compensated respiratory acidosis). The base excess is increased (>2 mEq/L) in these cases.

These relationships are shown diagrammatically in **Figure 2.10**. Contrast the steep slope of the line for acute CO_2 retention (A) with the shallow slope of the line for chronic hypercapnia (B). Note also that a patient with acute hypoventilation whose P_{CO_2} is maintained over 2 or 3 days moves toward the chronic line as the kidney conserves bicarbonate (point *A* to point *C*). Conversely, a patient with COPD with long-standing CO_2 retention who develops an acute chest infection with worsening of ventilation–perfusion relationships may move rapidly from point *B* to point *C*, that is, parallel to line *A*. However, if he is then mechanically ventilated, he may move back to point *B*, or even beyond.

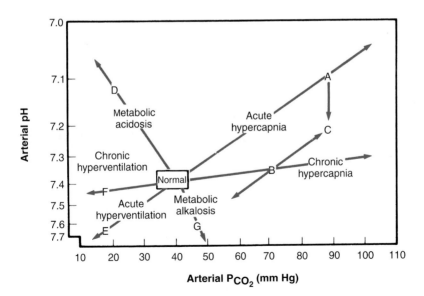

Figure 2.10. Arterial pH–P_{CO_2} relationships in various types of acid–base disturbances. (Modified from Flenley DC. Another nonlogarithmic acid–base diagram? *Lancet* 1971;1:961–965.)

Metabolic Acidosis
This is caused by a primary fall in the numerator (HCO₃⁻) of the Henderson-Hasselbalch equation, an example being diabetic ketoacidosis. Uncompensated metabolic acidosis would be indicated by a vertical upward movement on Figure 2.10, but in practice, the fall in arterial pH stimulates the peripheral chemoreceptors, increasing the ventilation and lowering the P_{CO_2}. As a result, the pH and P_{CO_2} move along line *D*.

Lactic acidosis is another form of metabolic acidosis, and this may complicate severe acute respiratory or cardiac failure as a consequence of tissue hypoxia. If such a patient is mechanically ventilated, the pH remains below 7.4 when the P_{CO_2} is returned to normal.

Alkalosis
Alkalosis (or alkalemia) results from an increase in arterial pH.

Respiratory Alkalosis
This is seen in acute hyperventilation where the pH rises, as shown by line *E* in Figure 2.10. If the hyperventilation is maintained, for example, at high altitude, compensated respiratory alkalosis is seen, with a return of the pH toward normal as the kidney excretes bicarbonate, a movement from point *E* to point *F* in Figure 2.10.

Metabolic Alkalosis
This is seen in disorders such as severe prolonged vomiting when the plasma bicarbonate concentration rises, as shown by *G* in Figure 2.10. Usually, there is no respiratory compensation but sometimes the P_{CO_2} rises slightly. Metabolic alkalosis also occurs when a patient with long-standing lung disease and compensated respiratory acidosis is ventilated too vigorously, thus bringing the P_{CO_2} rapidly to nearly 40 mm Hg (line *B* to *G*).

Four Types of Acid–Base Disturbance

$$pH = pK + \log\frac{(HCO_3^-)}{0.03\, P_{CO_2}}$$

	Primary	Compensation
Acidosis		
Respiratory	P_{CO_2} ↑	HCO_3^-↑
Metabolic	HCO_3^-↓	P_{CO_2} ↓
Alkalosis		
Respiratory	P_{CO_2} ↓	HCO_3^-↓
Metabolic	HCO_3^-↑	Often none

DIFFUSING CAPACITY

So far, this chapter on gas exchange has been devoted to arterial blood gases and their significance. However, this is a convenient place to discuss another common test of gas exchange—the diffusing capacity of the lung for carbon monoxide.

Measurement of Diffusing Capacity

The most popular method of measuring the diffusing capacity (D_{CO}) is the single-breath method **(Figure 2.11)**. The patient takes a vital capacity breath of 0.3% CO and 10% helium, holds his breath for 10 seconds, and then exhales. The first 750 mL of gas is discarded because of dead space contamination, and the next liter is collected and analyzed. The helium indicates the dilution of the inspired gas with alveolar gas and thus gives the initial alveolar P_{CO}. On the assumption that the CO is lost from alveolar gas in proportion to the P_{CO} during breath-holding, the diffusing capacity is calculated as the volume of CO taken up per minute per mm Hg alveolar P_{CO}.

Causes of Reduced Diffusing Capacity

Carbon monoxide is used to measure diffusing capacity because when it is inhaled in low concentrations, the partial pressure in the pulmonary capillary blood remains extremely low in relation to the alveolar value. As a result,

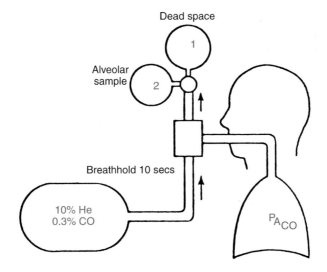

Figure 2.11. Measurement of the diffusing capacity for carbon monoxide by the single-breath method. The subject takes a single breath of 0.3% CO with 10% helium, holds his or her breath for 10 seconds, and then exhales. The first 750 mL is discarded, and then an alveolar sample is collected and analyzed.

CO is taken up by the blood all along the capillary (contrast the time course of O_2 shown in Figure 2.4). Thus, the uptake of CO is determined by the *diffusion properties* of the blood–gas barrier and the *rate of combination* of CO with blood.

The diffusion properties of the alveolar membrane depend on its thickness and area. Thus, the diffusing capacity is reduced by diseases in which the thickness is increased, including diffuse interstitial fibrosis, sarcoidosis, and asbestosis (Figure 2.5). It is also reduced when the surface area of the blood–gas barrier is reduced, for example, by pneumonectomy. The fall in diffusing capacity that occurs in emphysema is partly caused by the loss of alveolar walls and capillaries (however, see below).

The rate of combination of CO with blood is reduced when the number of red cells in the capillaries is reduced. This occurs in anemia and in diseases that reduce the capillary blood volume, such as pulmonary embolism. It is possible to separate the membrane and blood component of the diffusing capacity by making the measurement at a high and normal alveolar P_{O_2} (see *West's Respiratory Physiology: The Essentials.* 10th ed. pp. 34–37).

Interpretation of Diffusing Capacity

In many patients in whom the measured diffusing capacity is low, the interpretation is uncertain. The reason is the unevenness of ventilation, blood flow, and diffusion properties throughout the diseased lung. We know that such lungs tend to empty unevenly (see Figure 1.11), so that the liter of expired gas that is analyzed for CO (Figure 2.11) is probably not representative of the whole lung.

For this reason, the diffusing capacity is sometimes referred to as the *transfer factor* (especially in Europe) to emphasize that it is more a measure of the lung's overall ability to transfer gas into the blood than a specific test of diffusion characteristics. In spite of this uncertainty of interpretation, the test has a definite place in the pulmonary function laboratory and is frequently useful in assessing the severity and type of lung disease.

Causes of Reduced Diffusing Capacity for Carbon Monoxide

Blood–gas barrier
   Thickened in interstitial lung disease
   Area is reduced in emphysema, pneumonectomy
Capillary blood
   Volume reduced in pulmonary embolism
   Concentration of red cells reduced in anemia

KEY CONCEPTS

1. The measurement of arterial blood gases (P_{O_2}, P_{CO_2}, pH) is relatively simple with modern equipment and is essential in the treatment of patients with respiratory failure.

2. The four causes of hypoxemia are hypoventilation, diffusion impairment, shunt, and ventilation–perfusion inequality. The last is by far the most common cause.

3. Ventilation–perfusion inequality interferes with the exchange of all gases by the lung including O_2 and CO_2. All patients with this condition have a reduced arterial P_{O_2}, but the P_{CO_2} may be normal if the amount of inspired gas to the alveoli is increased.

4. Acid–base abnormalities include respiratory or metabolic acidosis and respiratory or metabolic alkalosis. These cause characteristic changes in pH, P_{CO_2}, and plasma bicarbonate.

5. The diffusing capacity for carbon monoxide is a useful test of gas transfer by the lung.

CLINICAL VIGNETTE

During a period of heavy smoke in the air caused by brush fires in the mountains surrounding her home, a 60-year-old woman with a long smoking history comes to the emergency department complaining of 2 days of increasing dyspnea and cough productive of purulent sputum. She had been seen in the outpatient pulmonary clinic just 2 weeks earlier for regular follow-up of her chronic respiratory issues, and at that time she had no new complaints and her pulmonary function tests showed the following:

Parameter	Predicted	Prebron- chodilator	% Predicted	Postbron- chodilator	% Change
FVC (L)	3.9	3.2	82	3.3	3
FEV$_1$ (L)	3.1	1.3	42	1.4	8
FEV$_1$/FVC	0.79	0.41	51	0.38	48
TLC (L)	5.8	6.3	109	—	—
RV (L)	1.9	2.9	152	—	—
DLCO (mL/ min/mm Hg)	33.4	15.7	47	—	—

In the emergency department, her temperature is 37.5°C, heart rate 105, blood pressure 137/83, respiratory rate 24,

(continued)

CLINICAL VIGNETTE (Continued)

and S_pO_2 82% while breathing ambient air. On examination, she is talking in short 3- to 4-word sentences and using accessory muscles of respiration. She has diffuse expiratory wheezes and a prolonged expiratory phase. Her chest is resonant to percussion throughout with limited excursion of the diaphragm on inhalation. Her chest radiograph shows large lung fields, flattened hemidiaphragms, and no focal opacities, effusions, or cardiomegaly. An arterial blood gas is performed prior to placing her on supplemental oxygen and shows the following:

pH	Pa_{CO_2} (mm Hg)	Pa_{O_2} (mm Hg)	HCO_3^- (mEq/L)
7.27	58	50	27

In addition to giving her nebulized bronchodilators and intravenous corticosteroids, she is placed on noninvasive positive pressure ventilation through a tight-fitting mask after which her dyspnea decreases and she appears more comfortable.

Questions
- How can you relate the abnormalities on spirometry performed in clinic 2 weeks ago to the findings on exam in the emergency department?
- What information does the diffusion capacity for carbon monoxide provide about her lung function?
- How would you interpret her arterial blood gases?
- What is the cause of her hypoxemia at the time of her presentation to the emergency department?
- What change would you expect to see in her Pa_{CO_2} after she was started on noninvasive ventilation?

QUESTIONS

1. In peripheral capillaries, more oxygen can be unloaded from the blood to the tissues at a given P_{O_2} when:
   A. Blood temperature is reduced.
   B. P_{CO_2} is reduced.
   C. Blood pH is raised.
   D. Concentration of 2,3-DPG in the red cell is raised.
   E. Hydrogen ion concentration is reduced.

2. A patient with chronic pulmonary disease undergoes emergency surgery. Postoperatively, the arterial P_{O_2}, P_{CO_2}, and pH are 50 mm Hg, 50 mm Hg, and 7.20, respectively. How would the acid–base status be best described?
  A. Mixed respiratory and metabolic acidosis
  B. Uncompensated respiratory acidosis
  C. Fully compensated respiratory acidosis
  D. Uncompensated metabolic acidosis
  E. Fully compensated metabolic acidosis

3. Which of the following mechanisms of hypoxemia will prevent the arterial P_{O_2} reaching the expected level if the subject is given 100% oxygen to breathe?
  A. Hypoventilation
  B. Diffusion impairment
  C. Ventilation–perfusion inequality
  D. Shunt
  E. Residence at high altitude

4. In a normal person, doubling the diffusing capacity would be expected to:
  A. Increase arterial P_{O_2} during moderate exercise.
  B. Increase the uptake of halothane given during anesthesia.
  C. Decrease arterial P_{CO_2} during resting breathing.
  D. Increase resting oxygen uptake when the subject breathes air.
  E. Increase maximal oxygen uptake at extreme altitude.

5. The laboratory provides the following report on a patient's arterial blood: pH, 7.25; P_{CO_2}, 32 mm Hg; and HCO_3^- concentration, 25 mmol/L. You conclude that there is:
  A. Respiratory alkalosis with metabolic compensation.
  B. Acute respiratory acidosis.
  C. Metabolic acidosis with respiratory compensation.
  D. Metabolic alkalosis with respiratory compensation.
  E. A laboratory error.

6. A 56-year-old woman complains of dyspnea on exertion over a several month period. Her pulmonary function tests show an FEV_1/FVC ratio of 0.83, TLC 85% predicted, and a diffusing capacity for carbon monoxide of 53% predicted. A chest radiograph shows a normal heart size and no focal opacities or effusions. A CT pulmonary angiogram shows no evidence of pulmonary embolism. Which of the following diagnoses could account for the findings on her evaluation thus far?
  A. Asthma
  B. Chronic obstructive pulmonary disease
  C. Idiopathic pulmonary fibrosis
  D. Iron deficiency anemia
  E. Sarcoidosis

7. A 48-year-old man is brought into the emergency department with decreased level of consciousness. An arterial blood gas shows pH 7.25, Pa_{CO_2} 25, Pa_{O_2} 62, and HCO_3^- 15. Which of the following could account for the observed abnormalities on his blood gases?
   A. Chronic obstructive pulmonary disease exacerbation
   B. Diabetic ketoacidosis
   C. Gastroenteritis with severe vomiting
   D. Morbid obesity
   E. Opiate overdose

8. A healthy 21-year-old woman flies from Lima (sea level) to Cuzco, Peru (altitude 3,350 m), on her way to Machu Picchu. Which of the following would likely occur immediately following arrival at Cuzco?
   A. Decreased diffusing capacity for carbon monoxide
   B. Decreased rate of rise of P_{O_2} in the pulmonary capillary
   C. Hypoventilation
   D. Increased shunt ($\dot{Q}_S/\dot{Q}_T$)
   E. Metabolic alkalosis

9. Which of the following could account for movement from condition A to condition B in the figure below?

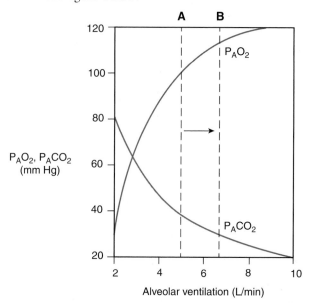

A. Anxiety attack
B. COPD exacerbation
C. Guillain-Barré syndrome
D. Opiate overdose
E. Poliomyelitis

10. A 61-year-old woman with chronic obstructive pulmonary disease comes to a hospital at sea level after several days of worsening dyspnea and increasing cough and sputum production. A chest radiograph shows changes consistent with emphysema but no focal opacities. An arterial blood gas is obtained while she is breathing ambient air and reveals pH 7.41, Pa_{CO_2} 39, Pa_{O_2} 62, and HCO_3^- 23. Which of the following is the cause of her hypoxemia?

A. Diffusion impairment
B. Hypoventilation
C. Low $P_{I_{O_2}}$
D. Ventilation–perfusion inequality
E. Hypoventilation and ventilation perfusion inequality

OTHER TESTS

3

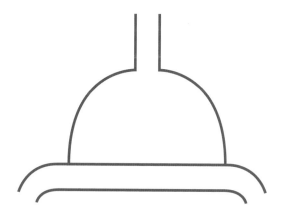

- **Static Lung Volumes**
  Measurement
  Interpretation
- **Lung Elasticity**
  Measurement
  Interpretation
- **Airway Resistance**
  Measurement
  Interpretation
- **Control of Ventilation**
  Measurement
  Interpretation
- **Exercise Tests**
  Measurement
  Interpretation
- **Dyspnea**
- **Topographic Differences of Lung Function**
  Measurement
  Interpretation
- **Value of Pulmonary Function Tests**

In Chapters 1 and 2, we concentrated on two simple but informative tests of pulmonary function: forced expiration and arterial blood gases. In this chapter, we briefly consider some other ways of measuring lung function. Of the large number of possible tests that have been introduced from time to time, we address only the most useful here and emphasize the principles rather than the details of their use.

STATIC LUNG VOLUMES

Measurement

The measurement of the vital capacity with a simple spirometer was described in Chapter 1 (Figure 1.1). This equipment can also be used to obtain the tidal volume, vital capacity, and expiratory reserve volume (functional residual capacity [FRC] minus the residual volume [RV]). However, the residual volume, functional residual capacity, and total lung capacity require additional measurements.

The FRC can be measured with a body plethysmograph, which is essentially a large airtight box in which the patient sits. (See *West's Respiratory Physiology: The Essentials.* 10th ed. p. 17.) The mouthpiece is obstructed, and the patient is instructed to make a rapid inspiratory effort. As he expands the gas volume in the lungs, the air in the plethysmograph is compressed slightly, and its pressure rises. By applying Boyle's law, the lung volume can be obtained. Another method is to use the helium dilution technique, in which a spirometer of known volume and helium concentration is connected to the patient in a closed circuit. From the degree of dilution of the helium, the unknown lung volume can be calculated. The residual volume can be derived from the FRC by subtracting the expiratory reserve volume.

Interpretation

The FRC and RV are typically increased in diseases in which there is an increased airway resistance, for example, emphysema, chronic bronchitis, and asthma. Indeed, at one time, an elevated RV was regarded as an essential feature of emphysema. The RV is raised in these conditions because airway closure occurs at an abnormally high lung volume.

A reduced FRC and RV are often seen in patients with reduced lung compliance, for example, in diffuse interstitial fibrosis. In this case, the lung is stiff and tends to recoil to a smaller resting volume.

If the FRC is measured by both the plethysmographic and gas dilution methods, a comparison of the two results is often informative. The plethysmographic method measures all the gas in the lung. However, the dilution technique "sees" only those regions of the lung that communicate with the mouth. Therefore, regions behind closed airways (e.g., some cysts and blebs) result in a higher value for the plethysmographic than for the dilution procedure. The same disparity is often seen in patients with chronic obstructive pulmonary disease, probably because some areas are so poorly ventilated that they do not equilibrate in the time allowed.

LUNG ELASTICITY

Measurement

The pressure–volume curve of the lung requires knowledge of the pressures both in the airways and around the lung (see *West's Respiratory Physiology: The Essentials*. 10th ed. p. 111). A good estimate of the latter can be obtained from the esophageal pressure. A small balloon at the end of a catheter is passed down through the nose or mouth to the lower esophagus, and the difference between the mouth and esophageal pressures is recorded as the patient exhales in steps of 1 liter from total lung capacity (TLC) to RV. The resulting pressure–volume curve is not linear **(Figure 3.1)**, so that a single value for its slope (compliance) can be misleading. However, the compliance is sometimes reported for the liter above FRC measured on the descending limb of the pressure–volume curve.

The pressure–volume curve is often reported using the percentage of predicted TLC on the vertical axis rather than using the actual lung volume in liters (Figure 3.1). This procedure helps to allow for differences in body size and reduces the variability of the results.

Interpretation

Elastic recoil is *reduced* in patients with emphysema. Figure 3.1 shows that the pressure–volume curve is displaced to the left and has a steeper slope in this condition as a result of the destruction of the alveolar walls (see also Figures 4.2, 4.3, and 4.5) and the consequent disorganization of elastic tissue.

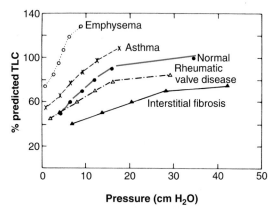

Figure 3.1. Pressure–volume curves of the lung. Note that the curves for emphysema and asthma (during an attack) are shifted upward and to the left, whereas those for rheumatic valve disease and interstitial fibrosis are flattened. (From Bates DV, Macklem PT, Christie RV. *Respiratory Function in Disease*. 2nd ed. Philadelphia, PA: WB Saunders, 1971.)

The change in compliance is not reversible. The pressure–volume curve is also typically shifted to the left in patients who are having an asthma attack, but the change is reversible in some patients. The reasons for this shift are unclear. Increasing age also tends to reduce elastic recoil.

Some Conditions Affecting Lung Elasticity	
Elastic recoil is *reduced* in	emphysema
	some patients with asthma
Elastic recoil is *increased* by	interstitial fibrosis
	interstitial edema

Elastic recoil is *increased* in interstitial fibrosis, which results in the deposition of fibrous tissue in the alveolar walls (see Figures 2.5 and 5.3), thus reducing the lung's distensibility. Elastic recoil also tends to increase in patients with rheumatic heart disease who have a raised pulmonary capillary pressure and some interstitial edema. However, note that measurements of the pressure–volume curve show considerable variability, and the neat results shown in Figure 3.1 are based on mean values from many patients.

AIRWAY RESISTANCE

Measurement

Airway resistance is measured as the pressure difference between the alveoli and the mouth divided by the flow rate. Alveolar pressure can only be measured indirectly: one way to do this is with a body plethysmograph. (See *West's Respiratory Physiology: The Essentials*. 10th ed. p. 192.) The subject sits in an airtight box and pants through a flow meter. The alveolar pressure can be deduced from the pressure changes in the plethysmograph because, when the alveolar gas is compressed, the plethysmograph gas volume increases slightly, causing a fall in pressure. This method has the advantage that lung volume can be measured easily almost simultaneously. **Figure 3.2** shows the effect of cigarette smoking on airway resistance, here expressed as its reciprocal, *conductance*.

Interpretation

Airway resistance is reduced by an increase in lung volume because the expanding parenchyma exerts traction on the airway walls. Thus, any measurement of airway resistance must be related to the lung volume. Note that the small peripheral airways normally contribute little to overall resistance because

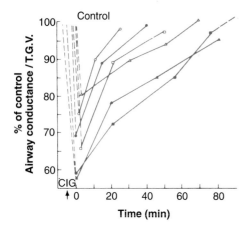

Figure 3.2. Effect of cigarette smoking on airway conductance as measured in the body plethysmograph. The ordinate shows conductance related to thoracic gas volume. (From Nadel JA, Comroe Jr, JH. Acute effects of inhalation of cigarette smoke on airway conductance. *J Appl Physiol* 1961;16:713–716.)

there are so many arranged in parallel. For this reason, special tests have been devised to try to detect early changes in small airways. These changes include the flow rate during the latter part of the flow–volume curve (see Figure 1.8) and closing volume (see Figure 1.10).

Some Conditions Affecting Airway Resistance

Resistance is *increased* by	chronic bronchitis
	asthma
	emphysema
	inhaled irritants (e.g., cigarette smoke)
Resistance is *decreased* by	increased lung volume

Airway resistance is *increased* in chronic bronchitis and emphysema. In chronic bronchitis, the lumen of a typical airway contains excessive secretions and the wall is thickened by mucous gland hyperplasia and edema (see Figure 4.6). In emphysema, many of the airways lose the radical traction of the tissue surrounding them because of destruction of the alveolar walls (see Figures 4.1 and 4.2). As a result, their resistance may not increase much during quiet breathing (it may be nearly normal), but with any exertion, dynamic compression (see Figure 1.6) quickly occurs on expiration, and resistance rises strikingly. Such patients often show a reasonably high flow rate early in expiration, but this abruptly drops to low values as flow limitation occurs (see the flow–volume curve in Figure 1.8). Recall that the driving pressure under these conditions is the static recoil pressure of the lung (see Figure 1.6), which is reduced in emphysema (Figure 3.1).

Airway resistance is also increased in patients with bronchial asthma. Here, the factors include bronchial smooth muscle contraction and hypertrophy, increased mucous production, and edema of the airway walls (see Figure 4.14). The resistance may be high during attacks, especially in relation to lung volume, which is frequently greatly increased. The resistance is reduced by bronchodilator drugs such as β2-agonists. Even during periods of remission when the patient is asymptomatic, airway resistance is often raised.

Tracheal obstruction increases airway resistance. This may be caused by compression from outside, for example, an enlarged thyroid, or by intrinsic narrowing caused by scarring or a tumor (fixed obstruction). An important feature is that the obstruction is usually apparent during *inspiration* and it can be detected on an inspiratory flow–volume curve (see Figure 1.9). In addition, an audible stridor may be present.

CONTROL OF VENTILATION

Measurement

The ventilatory response to carbon dioxide can be measured with a rebreathing technique. A small bag is filled with a mixture of 6–7% CO_2 in oxygen, and the patient rebreathes from this over a period of several minutes. The bag P_{CO_2} increases at the rate of 4 to 6 mm Hg/min because of the CO_2 being produced from the tissues, and thus, the change in ventilation per mm Hg increase in P_{CO_2} can be determined.

The ventilatory response to hypoxia can be measured in a similar way. In this instance, the bag is filled with 24% O_2, 7% CO_2, and the balance with N_2. During rebreathing, the P_{CO_2} is monitored and held constant by means of a variable bypass and CO_2 absorber. As the oxygen is taken up, the increase in ventilation is related to the P_{O_2} in the bag and lungs.

Both these techniques give information about the overall ventilatory response to CO_2 or hypoxemia, but they do not differentiate between patients who *will not* breathe because of central nervous system or neuromuscular inadequacy and those who *cannot* breathe because of mechanical abnormalities of the chest or muscles of respiration. To make this distinction between those who "won't" and those who "can't" breathe, the mechanical work done during inspiration can be measured. To accomplish this, the esophageal pressure is recorded with tidal volume, and the area of the pressure–volume loop is obtained. (See *West's Respiratory Physiology: The Essentials.* 10th ed. pp. 134–135.) Inspiratory work recorded in this way is one useful measure of the neural output of the respiratory center.

Interpretation

The ventilatory response to CO_2 is depressed by sleep, narcotic drugs and genetic factors. An important question is why some patients with chronic pulmonary disease develop CO_2 retention and others do not. In this context, considerable differences of CO_2 response exist among individuals, and it has been suggested that the course of patients with chronic respiratory disease may be related to this factor. Thus, patients who respond strongly to a rise in P_{CO_2} may be more distressed by dyspnea, whereas those who respond weakly may allow their P_{CO_2} to rise and they succumb to respiratory failure. A similar phenomenon of CO_2 retention and depressed ventilatory responses to CO_2 is seen in some morbidly obese individuals.

The factors that affect the ventilatory response to hypoxia are less clearly understood. However, the response is reduced in many persons who have been hypoxemic since birth, such as those born at high altitude or with cyanotic congenital heart disease. The hypoxic ventilatory response tends to be preserved during sleep.

EXERCISE TESTS

Measurement

The normal lung has enormous reserves of function at rest. For example, the O_2 uptake and CO_2 output can be increased 10-fold or more when a normal person exercises, and these increases occur without a fall in arterial P_{O_2} or a rise in P_{CO_2}. Therefore, to reveal minor dysfunction, the stress of exercise is often useful.

Another reason for exercise testing is to assess disability. Patients vary considerably in their own assessment of the amount of activity they can do, and an objective measurement on a treadmill, stationary bicycle, or a walk along a hallway can be revealing. Occasionally, exercise tests are diagnostic, for example, in exercise-induced asthma and in myocardial ischemia causing angina. Exercise tests can help evaluate the primary system limiting exercise when simpler tests such as spirometry or echocardiography are not revealing.

The variables that are often measured during exercise include work load, total ventilation, respiratory frequency, tidal volume, heart rate, ECG, blood pressure, O_2 uptake, CO_2 output, arterial P_{O_2}, P_{CO_2}, and pH. More specialized measurements, such as diffusing capacity, cardiac output, and blood lactate concentration, are sometimes made. Abnormal gas exchange can be characterized by the physiologic dead space and shunt as at rest.

Some investigators take special note of the respiratory exchange ratio (R) as the exercise level is increased. This can be calculated on a continuous basis using current breath-by-breath exercise systems. When the patient reaches the limit of his or her steady-state aerobic exercise (sometimes called the *anaerobic threshold* or *ventilatory threshold*), the R rises more rapidly. This is caused by an increase in the CO_2 production secondary to the liberation of lactic acid from the hypoxic muscles. The hydrogen ions react with bicarbonate and lead to an increase in CO_2 excretion above that produced by aerobic metabolism. The fall in pH provides an additional stimulus to breathing.

Less formal exercise tests (so-called field exercise tests) can also be informative. One is the 6-minute walk test (6MWT), in which the patient is asked to walk as far as possible along a corridor or other flat terrain for 6 minutes. The result is expressed in meters covered and has the advantage that the test simulates real-life conditions. The results often improve with practice. Other field tests include the incremental shuttle walk test, in which the patient walks around two cones placed 10 m apart at a steadily increasing speed set by beeps from an audiotape device, and the endurance shuttle walk test in which the individual walks as long as tolerated at a constant preset pace. These field tests are only of utility in patients with limited exercise capacity and are not useful for assessing exercise responses in fit individuals.

Interpretation

In most instances, the interpretation of the tests during exercise is similar to that of tests done at rest except that exercise exaggerates the abnormalities. For example, a patient with interstitial lung disease who has a marginally reduced diffusing capacity at rest may show almost no increase on exercise (an abnormal result), with a marked fall in arterial P_{O_2}, a relatively small rise in cardiac output, and perhaps striking dyspnea. **Figure 3.3B** shows the

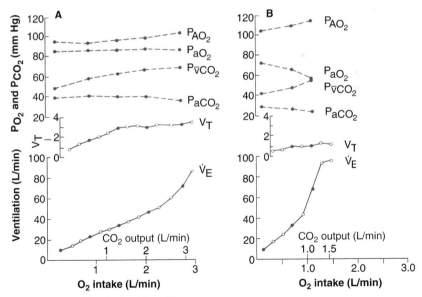

Figure 3.3. Results obtained during exercise testing. A. Normal pattern. **B.** Results in a patient with hypersensitivity pneumonitis. Note the restricted work level evidenced by the limited O_2 intake, the excessive ventilation for the O_2 intake, and the marked fall in arterial P_{O_2}. (From Jones NL. Exercise testing in pulmonary evaluation. *N Engl J Med* 1975;293:541–544, 647–650.)

exercise response of a patient with hypersensitivity pneumonitis. Note the rapid increase in ventilation at relatively low work levels and the fall in arterial P_{O_2} and P_{CO_2}.

Sometimes, it is possible to identify the chief factor limiting exercise in a patient with mixed disease. For example, patients who have both heart and lung disease present a common problem. Exercise testing may reveal that at a patient's maximum work load, there is abnormal pulmonary gas exchange with a high physiologic dead space and shunt, suggesting that the patient's lung is the weak link. Alternatively, the cardiac output may respond poorly to exercise, thus suggesting heart disease as the chief culprit. Sometimes, however, the interpretation is not clear-cut.

DYSPNEA

Dyspnea refers to the sensation of difficulty with breathing, and it should be distinguished from simple tachypnea (rapid breathing) or hyperpnea (increased ventilation). Because dyspnea is a subjective phenomenon, it is difficult to measure, and the factors responsible for it are poorly understood. Broadly speaking, dyspnea occurs when the *demand for ventilation* is out of proportion to the patient's *ability to respond* to that demand. As a result, breathing becomes difficult, uncomfortable, or labored.

An *increased demand for ventilation* is often caused by changes in the blood gases and pH level. High ventilations on exercise are common in patients with inefficient pulmonary gas exchange, especially those with large physiologic dead spaces, who tend to develop CO_2 retention and acidosis unless they achieve high ventilations. Another important factor is stimulation of intrapulmonary receptors. This factor presumably explains the high exercise ventilations in many patients with interstitial lung disease, possibly as a result of stimulation of the juxtacapillary (J) receptors (Figure 3.3B).

A *reduced ability to respond* to the ventilatory needs is generally caused by abnormal mechanics of the lung or chest wall. Frequently, increased airway resistance is the problem, as in asthma, but other causes include a stiff chest wall, as in kyphoscoliosis.

The assessment of dyspnea is difficult. One way is to ask the patient to indicate his or her perceived feeling of dyspnea on a linear scale from 1 to 10, with 1 being the lowest and 10 the highest. This type of measurement is especially useful before and after an intervention such as treatment with a bronchodilator. Exercise tolerance is often determined from a standard questionnaire that grades breathlessness according to how far the patient can walk on the level or go upstairs without pausing for breath. The Borg Dyspnea Scale is an example of a questionnaire commonly used for this purpose. Occasionally, in an attempt to obtain an index of dyspnea, ventilation is measured at a standard level of exercise and is then related to the patient's maximum voluntary ventilation. However, dyspnea is something that only the patient feels; as such, it cannot be measured objectively.

TOPOGRAPHIC DIFFERENCES OF LUNG FUNCTION

Measurement

The regional distribution of blood flow and ventilation in the lung can be measured with radioactive substances (see *West's Respiratory Physiology: The Essentials*. 10th ed. pp. 24, 49). One method of detecting areas of absent blood flow is by injecting albumin aggregates labeled with radioactive technetium. An image of the radioactivity is then made with a gamma camera, and "cold" areas containing no activity are readily apparent. The distribution of blood flow can also be obtained from an intravenous injection of radioactive xenon or other gas dissolved in saline. When the gas reaches the pulmonary capillaries, it is evolved into the alveolar gas, and the radiation can be detected by a gamma camera. This method has the advantage of giving blood flow per unit volume of lung.

The distribution of ventilation can be measured in a similar way, except that the gas is inhaled into the alveoli from a spirometer. Either a single inspiration or a wash-in over a series of breaths can be recorded. This method of assessing ventilation can be combined with the technetium-labeled albumin technique described above to diagnose pulmonary embolism, although this approach has since been supplanted by CT pulmonary angiography as the diagnostic method of choice.

Interpretation

The distribution of blood flow in the upright lung is uneven, being much greater at the base than at the apex **(Figure 3.4)**. The differences are caused by gravity and can be explained by the relationships between the pulmonary arterial, venous, and alveolar pressures. (See *West's Respiratory Physiology: The Essentials*. 10th ed. p. 50.) Exercise results in a more uniform distribution because of the increase in pulmonary arterial pressure; the same result is found in disease conditions such as pulmonary hypertension and right-to-left cardiac shunts. Localized lung disease, for example, a bleb or a bulla, or area of fibrosis, frequently decreases regional blood flow.

The distribution of ventilation is also gravity dependent, and normally, the ventilation to the base exceeds that to the apex. The explanation is the distortion that the lung suffers because of gravity and the larger

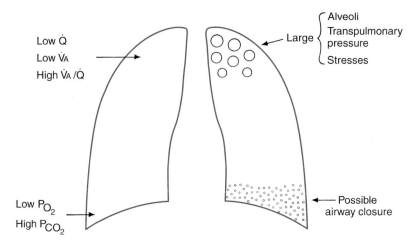

Low $\dot{Q}$
Low $\dot{V}_A$
High $\dot{V}_A/\dot{Q}$

Large — Alveoli, Transpulmonary pressure, Stresses

Low P_{O_2}
High P_{CO_2}

Possible airway closure

Figure 3.4. Regional differences of structure and function in the upright lung.

transpulmonary pressure at the apex compared with the base. (See *West's Respiratory Physiology: The Essentials.* 10th ed. p. 118.) Localized lung disease, for example, a bulla, usually reduces the ventilation in that area. In generalized lung diseases—such as asthma, chronic bronchitis, emphysema, and interstitial fibrosis—areas of reduced ventilation and blood flow can frequently be detected.

Healthy people show a reversal of the normal pattern of ventilation if they inhale a small amount of radioactive gas from residual volume. The reason is that the airways at the base of the lung are closed under these conditions because intrapleural pressure actually rises above airway pressure. The same pattern may occur at FRC in older subjects because the lower-zone airways close at an abnormally high lung volume. Similar findings may be seen in patients with emphysema, interstitial edema, and obesity. All these conditions exaggerate airway closure at the base of the lung.

Other regional differences of structure and function also occur. The gravity-induced distortion of the upright lung causes the alveoli at the apex to be larger than those at the base. These larger alveoli are also associated with greater mechanical stresses that may play a role in the development of some diseases, such as centriacinar emphysema (see Figure 4.5A) and spontaneous pneumothorax.

VALUE OF PULMONARY FUNCTION TESTS

Because this book is about the function of diseased lungs, it is natural that we should start with pulmonary function tests. However, it is important to recognize that these tests have a limited role in clinical practice. They are rarely useful in making a specific diagnosis; rather, they provide supporting information that is added to that obtained from the clinical history, physical examination, chest imaging, and laboratory tests. Lung function tests are particularly valuable in following the progress of a patient, for example, assessing the efficacy of bronchodilator therapy in a patient with asthma or monitoring patients for immune rejection after lung transplantation. They are also useful in assessing patients prior to surgical resection of portions of the lung, determining disability for purposes of workers' compensation, and estimating the prevalence of disease in a community, for example, in a coal mine or an asbestos factory. Lung function tests are occasionally within normal limits despite obvious generalized lung diseases.

As has been emphasized, spirometry gives useful information with simple equipment. Arterial blood gases are more difficult to measure, but the data may be lifesaving for patients with respiratory failure. The value of the other tests depends largely on the clinical problem, and whether they are worth doing is related to the facilities of the pulmonary function laboratory, the expense, and the likelihood that they will give useful information.

KEY CONCEPTS

1. Lung elastic recoil is reduced in emphysema and some patients with asthma. It is increased in interstitial fibrosis and slightly in interstitial edema.

2. Airway resistance is increased in chronic bronchitis, emphysema, and asthma. It is reduced by increasing lung volume. Fixed tracheal obstruction increases both inspiratory and expiratory resistance.

3. The control of ventilation by increased P_{CO_2} and reduced P_{O_2} varies greatly among people and may affect the clinical pattern of patients with severe chronic obstructive pulmonary disease and morbid obesity.

4. The lung at rest has enormous reserves of function, and valuable information can therefore often be obtained during exercise that stresses gas exchange.

5. Dyspnea is a common, important symptom in many lung diseases but can be truly assessed only by the patient.

CLINICAL VIGNETTE

A 30-year-old woman is referred to the pulmonary clinic for evaluation of 6 months of worsening dyspnea on exertion and a nonproductive cough. She had not had fevers, weight loss, or chest pain but had to stop her weekly dance classes due to dyspnea. She is a life-long nonsmoker and has several pets at home including a dog, a cat, and a cockatiel she received one year ago from a friend who had to give it up due to a respiratory disorder. In the clinic, she is afebrile and has a normal heart rate, blood pressure, and respiratory rate and an S_PO_2 of 96% breathing ambient air. The only noteworthy finding on her exam is the presence of fine end-inspiratory crackles in the bilateral lower lung zones. A plain chest radiograph shows faint bilateral opacities while a follow-up chest CT scan shows diffuse "ground-glass opacities" consistent with an alveolar-filling process. Pulmonary function tests show the following:

Parameter	Predicted	Prebron- chodilator	% Predicted	Postbron- chodilator	% Change
FVC (L)	4.37	1.73	40	1.79	4
FEV₁ (L)	3.65	1.57	43	1.58	0
FEV₁/FVC	0.84	0.91	108	0.88	−3
TLC (L)	6.12	2.68	44	—	—
DLCO (mL/min/mm Hg)	32.19	15.13	47	—	—

Questions
- What changes would you expect to see in her FRC and RV?
- If you were able to obtain estimates of pleural pressure using a catheter inserted through her nose into her esophagus, what changes would you expect to see in the pressure–volume curve for her lungs?
- How will her airway resistance compare to that of a healthy individual?
- What would you expect to happen to her P_{aO_2} during a cardiopulmonary exercise test?

QUESTIONS

1. In the upright human lung, which of the following is greater at the apex than the base?
   A. Blood flow
   B. Ventilation
   C. Alveolar P_{CO_2}
   D. Alveolar size
   E. Capillary blood volume

2. Airway resistance in a patient with asthma:
A. Is raised by increasing lung volume.
B. Is reduced by inhaling β_2-agonists.
C. Is increased by destruction of alveolar walls.
D. Is unaffected by secretions in the airways.
E. Is increased by loss of bronchial smooth muscle.

3. During an exercise test on a patient with mitral stenosis, it was found that the respiratory exchange ratio of expired gas rapidly rose above 1 at a low level of exercise. A likely reason is:
A. Abnormally high levels of lactate in the blood.
B. Abnormally low ventilation.
C. Abnormally high cardiac output.
D. Increased lung compliance.
E. Reduced diffusing capacity of the lung.

4. A 41-year-old woman complains of acute dyspnea and chest pain. She is sent for a ventilation–perfusion scan in which she inhales radiolabeled xenon and receives an injection of technetium-labeled macroaggregated albumin. Using a gamma camera, images are recorded that reflect the ventilation and perfusion throughout each lung. The ventilation images reveal a homogenous pattern of activity throughout the entirety of both lungs, while the perfusion images show a large area with no activity in the left lower lobe. Based on these results, what is the most likely cause of her dyspnea and chest pain?
A. Asthma exacerbation
B. Chronic obstructive pulmonary disease exacerbation
C. Myocardial infarction
D. Pneumothorax
E. Pulmonary embolism

5. A 65-year-old man with a long history of smoking presents with one year of worsening dyspnea on exertion. On auscultation, he has scattered expiratory musical sounds and a prolonged expiratory phase. A chest radiograph reveals large lung volumes, flattened diaphragms, and decreased lung markings in the apical regions, while spirometry shows a reduced FEV_1 and FVC and FEV_1/FVC of 0.62. Which of the following would you expect to observe on further pulmonary function testing?
A. Decreased total lung capacity
B. Decreased airway resistance
C. Decreased lung compliance
D. Increased diffusion capacity for carbon monoxide
E. Increased functional residual capacity

6. A 68-year-old woman undergoes pulmonary function testing as part of an evaluation for dyspnea and chronic cough. When lung volume measurements are obtained using both body plethysmography and helium dilution, the residual volume is found to be 0.6 liters higher when measured by plethysmography than when measured by helium dilution. Which of the following underlying diseases could account for this observation?
   A. Asbestosis
   B. Chronic obstructive pulmonary disease
   C. Heart Failure
   D. Idiopathic pulmonary fibrosis
   E. Neuromuscular disease

PART **TWO**

FUNCTION OF THE DISEASED LUNG

4 ■ **Obstructive Diseases**

5 ■ **Restrictive Diseases**

6 ■ **Vascular Diseases**

7 ■ **Environmental, Neoplastic, and Infectious Diseases**

This part is devoted to the patterns of abnormal function in some common types of lung disease.

OBSTRUCTIVE DISEASES

4

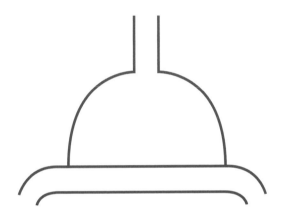

- **Airway Obstruction**
- **Chronic Obstructive Pulmonary Disease**
  Emphysema
    Pathology
    Types
    Pathogenesis
  Chronic Bronchitis
    Pathology
    Pathogenesis
  Clinical Features of Chronic Obstructive Pulmonary Disease
    Type A
    Type B
  Pulmonary Function
    Ventilatory Capacity and Mechanics
    Gas Exchange
    Pulmonary Circulation
    Control of Ventilation
    Changes in Early Disease
    Treatment of Patients with COPD

  Lung Volume Reduction Surgery

- **Asthma**
  Pathology
  Pathogenesis
  Clinical Features
  Bronchoactive Drugs
    β-Adrenergic Agonists
    Inhaled Corticosteroids
    Anticholinergics
    Cromolyn and Nedocromil
    Methylxanthines
    Leukotriene-Modifying Drugs
  Anti-IgE Therapy
  Pulmonary Function
    Ventilatory Capacity and Mechanics
    Gas Exchange

- **Localized Airway Obstruction**
  Tracheal Obstruction
  Bronchial Obstruction

Obstructive diseases of the lung are extremely common and remain an important cause of morbidity and mortality. While the distinctions among the various types of obstructive disease are blurred, giving rise to difficulties in definition and diagnosis, all of these diseases are characterized by airway obstruction.

AIRWAY OBSTRUCTION

Increased resistance to airflow can be caused by conditions (1) inside the lumen, (2) in the wall of the airway, and (3) in the peribronchial region **(Figure 4.1)**:

1. The lumen may be partially occluded by excessive secretions, such as in chronic bronchitis. Partial obstruction can also occur acutely in pulmonary edema or after aspiration of foreign material and, postoperatively, with retained secretions. Inhaled foreign bodies may cause localized partial or complete obstruction.
2. Causes in the wall of the airway include contraction of bronchial smooth muscle, as in asthma; hypertrophy of the mucous glands, as in chronic bronchitis (see Figure 4.6); and inflammation and edema of the wall, as in bronchitis and asthma.
3. Outside the airway, destruction of lung parenchyma may cause loss of radial traction and consequent narrowing, as in emphysema. A bronchus may also be compressed locally by an enlarged lymph node or neoplasm. Peribronchial edema can also cause narrowing (see Figure 6.5).

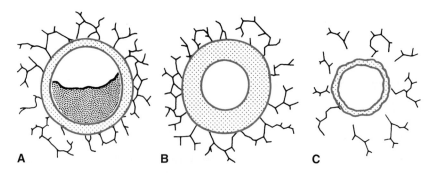

A   **B**   **C**

Figure 4.1. Mechanisms of airway obstruction. A. The lumen is partly blocked, for example, by excessive secretions. **B.** The airway wall is thickened, for example, by edema or hypertrophy of smooth muscle. **C.** The abnormality is outside the airway; in this example, the lung parenchyma is partly destroyed and the airway has narrowed because of the loss of radial traction.

CHRONIC OBSTRUCTIVE PULMONARY DISEASE

Chronic obstructive pulmonary disease (COPD) is caused by emphysema, chronic bronchitis, or a mixture of the two and is defined by the presence of airflow obstruction. Patients typically have increasing shortness of breath over several years, chronic cough, impaired exercise tolerance, as well as overinflated lungs and impaired gas exchange. It can often be difficult to determine to what extent patients have emphysema or chronic bronchitis, and the term "chronic obstructive pulmonary disease" is a convenient, nondescript label that avoids making an unwarranted diagnosis with inadequate data.

Emphysema

Emphysema is characterized by enlargement of the air spaces distal to the terminal bronchiole, with destruction of their walls. Note that this is an anatomic definition; in other words, the diagnosis is presumptive and based largely on radiologic findings in the living patient.

Pathology

A typical histologic appearance is shown in **Figure 4.2B**. Note that in contrast to the normal lung section in **Figure 4.2A**, the emphysematous lung shows loss of alveolar walls with consequent destruction of parts of the capillary bed. Strands of parenchyma that contain blood vessels can sometimes be seen coursing across large dilated airspaces. The small airways (less than 2 mm wide) are narrowed, tortuous, and reduced in number. In addition, they have thin, atrophied walls. There is also some loss of larger airways. The structural changes are well seen with the naked eye or hand lens in large slices of lung **(Figure 4.3)**.

Types

Various types of emphysema are recognized. The definition given earlier indicates that the disease affects the parenchyma distal to the terminal bronchiole. This unit is the *acinus*, but it may not be damaged uniformly. In *centriacinar emphysema*, the destruction is limited to the central part of the acinus, and the peripheral alveolar ducts and alveoli may escape unscathed **(Figure 4.4)**. By contrast, *panacinar emphysema* shows distension and destruction of the whole acinus. Occasionally, the disease is most marked in the lung adjacent to interlobular septa (paraseptal emphysema), while in other patients, large cystic areas or bullae develop (bullous emphysema).

Centriacinar and panacinar emphysema tend to have different topographic distributions. The former is typically most marked in the apex of the upper

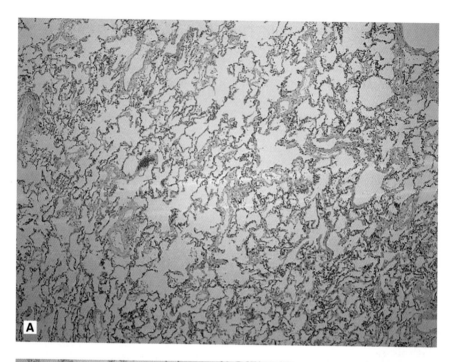

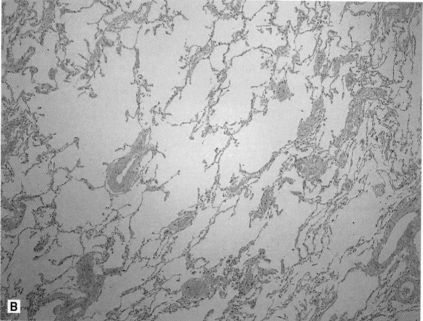

Figure 4.2. **Microscopic appearance of emphysematous lung. A.** Normal lung.
B. Loss of alveolar walls and consequent enlargement of airspaces (×4). (Image courtesy of Corinne Fligner, MD.)

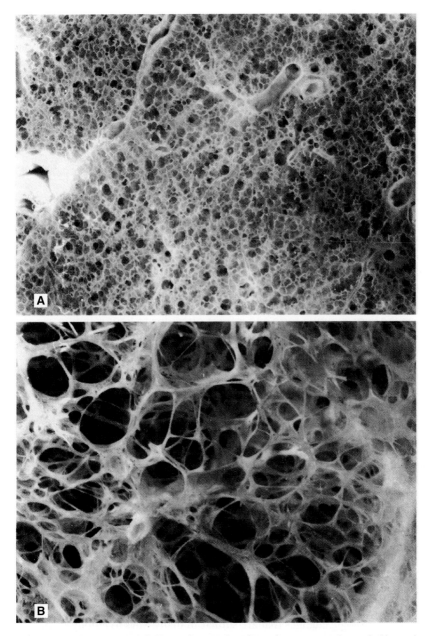

Figure 4.3. Appearance of slices of normal and emphysematous lung. A. Normal.
B. Panacinar emphysema (barium sulfate impregnation, ×14). (From Heard BE.
Pathology of Chronic Bronchitis and Emphysema. London, UK: Churchill, 1969.)

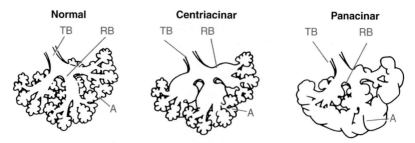

Normal   **Centriacinar**   **Panacinar**

TB   RB   TB   RB   TB   RB

A   A   A

Figure 4.4. **Centriacinar and panacinar emphysema.** In centriacinar emphysema, the destruction is confined to the terminal and respiratory bronchioles (*TB* and *RB*). In panacinar emphysema, the peripheral alveoli (*A*) are also involved.

lobe but spreads down the lung as the disease progresses **(Figure 4.5A)**. The predilection for the apex might reflect the higher mechanical stresses (see Figure 3.4), which predispose to structural failure of the alveolar walls. By contrast, panacinar emphysema has no regional preference or, possibly, is more common in the lower lobes. When emphysema is severe, it is difficult to distinguish the two types, and these may coexist in one lung. The centriacinar form is a very common form and is most often due to long-standing exposure to cigarette smoke. Mild forms apparently cause no dysfunction.

A severe form of panacinar emphysema can be seen in α_1-antitrypsin deficiency **(Figure 4.5B)**. The disease, which usually begins in the lower lobes, may become evident by the age of 40 years in patients who are homozygous for the Z gene, particularly in those who also smoke. Extrapulmonary manifestations may also be present in the liver, bowel, kidneys, and other organs. Therapy by replacement of α_1-antitrypsin is now available. Heterozygotes do not seem to be at risk, although this is not certain. Other variants of emphysema include unilateral emphysema (MacLeod's or Swyer-James syndrome), which causes a unilaterally hyperlucent chest radiograph.

Pathogenesis

One hypothesis is that excessive amounts of the enzyme lysosomal elastase are released from the neutrophils in the lung. This results in the destruction of elastin, an important structural protein of the lung. Neutrophil elastase also cleaves type IV collagen, and this molecule is important in determining the strength of the thin side of the pulmonary capillary and therefore the integrity of the alveolar wall. Animals that have had neutrophil elastase instilled into their airways develop histologic changes that are similar in many ways to emphysema.

Cigarette smoking is an important pathogenic factor and may work by stimulating macrophages to release neutrophil chemoattractants, such as C5a, or by reducing the activity of elastase inhibitors. In addition, many neutrophils are normally marginated (trapped) in the lung, and this process is exaggerated by cigarette smoking, which also activates trapped leucocytes.

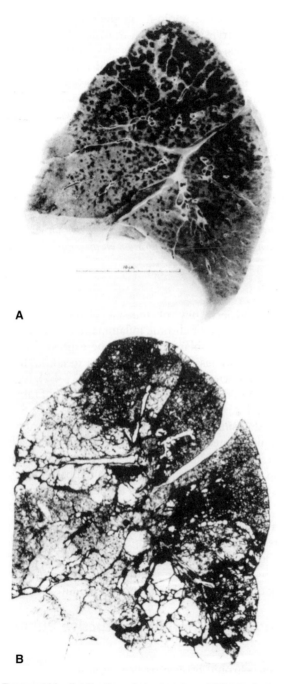

Figure 4.5. Topographic distribution of emphysema. A. The typical upper zone preference of centriacinar emphysema. **B.** The typical lower zone preference of emphysema caused by α_1-antitrypsin deficiency. (From Heard BE. *Pathology of Chronic Bronchitis and Emphysema.* London, UK: Churchill, 1969.)

This hypothesis puts the etiology on the same footing as that for the emphysema of α_1-antitrypsin deficiency, in which the mechanism is the lack of the antiprotease that normally inhibits elastase. One puzzle is why some heavy smokers do not develop the disease. Air pollution may play a role, as may hereditary factors, which are clearly important in α_1-antitrypsin deficiency. Smoke pollution from fuels, for example, from use of poorly ventilated wood-burning stoves indoors, is now also recognized as an important cause of COPD worldwide.

Chronic Bronchitis

This disease is characterized by excessive mucus production in the bronchial tree, sufficient to cause excessive expectoration of sputum. Note that this is a clinical definition (unlike the definition of emphysema). In practice, criteria for excessive expectoration are often laid down, for example, expectoration on most days for at least 3 months in the year for at least 2 successive years.

Pathology

The hallmark is hypertrophy of mucous glands in the large bronchi **(Figure 4.6)** and evidence of chronic inflammatory changes in the small airways. The mucous gland enlargement may be expressed as the gland–wall ratio, which is normally less than 0.4 but may exceed 0.7 in severe chronic bronchitis. This is known as the "Reid index" **(Figure 4.7)**. Excessive amounts of mucus are found in the airways, and semisolid plugs of mucus may occlude some small bronchi.

In addition, the small airways are narrowed and show inflammatory changes, including cellular infiltration and edema of the walls. Granulation tissue is present, bronchial smooth muscle increases, and peribronchial fibrosis may develop. There is evidence that the initial pathologic changes are in the small airways and that these progress to the larger bronchi.

Pathogenesis

Again, cigarette smoking is the chief culprit. Repeated exposure to this inhaled irritant results in chronic inflammation. If you hear a patient give a moist, fruity (or gurgling) cough, you can safely bet that he is a smoker. Air pollution caused by smog or industrial smoke is another definite factor.

Clinical Features of Chronic Obstructive Pulmonary Disease

As we have seen, chronic bronchitis is a clinical definition, and the diagnosis in the living patient can therefore be made confidently. However, a definitive diagnosis of emphysema requires histologic confirmation that is usually not available during life, although a combination of history, physical

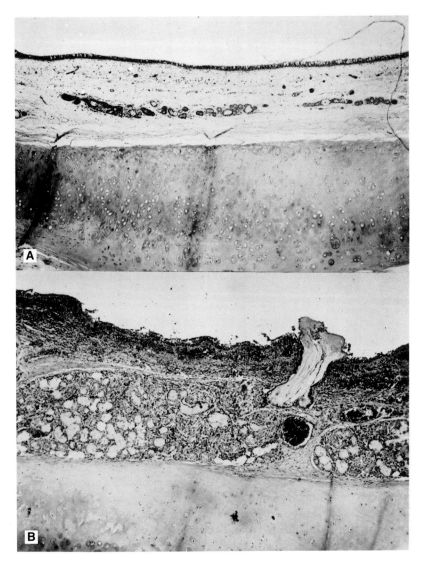

Figure 4.6. Histologic changes in chronic bronchitis. A. A normal bronchial wall. **B.** Bronchial wall of a patient with chronic bronchitis. Note the great hypertrophy of the mucous glands, the thickened submucosa, and the cellular infiltration (3× 60). Compare with the diagram of the bronchial wall in Figure 4.7. (From Thurlbeck WM. *Chronic Airflow Obstruction in Lung Disease.* Philadelphia, PA: WB Saunders, 1976.)

examination, and radiology (especially computed tomography [CT]) can give a high probability of the diagnosis. It follows that the amount of emphysema in a given patient is uncertain. This is why COPD remains a useful term.

Within the spectrum of COPD, two extremes of clinical presentation are recognized: type A and type B. At one time, it was thought that these types correlated

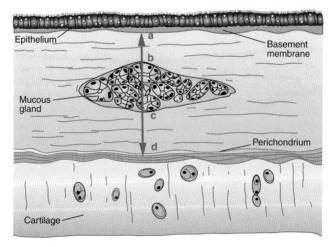

Figure 4.7. Structure of a normal bronchial wall. In chronic bronchitis, the thickness of the mucous glands increases and can be expressed as the Reid index given by (*b–c*)/(*a–d*). (From Thurlbeck WM. *Chronic Airflow Obstruction in Lung Disease.* Philadelphia, PA: WB Saunders, 1976.)

to some extent with the relative amounts of emphysema and chronic bronchitis, respectively, in the lung, but this view has been challenged. Nevertheless, it is still useful to describe two patterns of clinical presentation because they represent different pathophysiologies. In practice, most patients have features of both.

Type A
A typical presentation would be a man in his middle 50s who has had increasing shortness of breath for the last 3 or 4 years. Cough may be absent or may produce little white sputum. Physical examination reveals an asthenic build with evidence of recent weight loss. There is no cyanosis. The chest is overexpanded with quiet breath sounds and no adventitious sounds. The radiograph **(Figure 4.8B)** confirms the overinflation with low and flattened diaphragms, narrow mediastinum, and increased retrosternal translucency (between the sternum and the heart on the lateral view). In addition, the radiograph shows increased lucency, particularly in the apical lung zones, due to attenuation and narrowing of the peripheral pulmonary vessels. Additional information is available from computer tomography (CT). **Figure 4.9A** shows a normal lung using this imaging technique. **Figure 4.9B** shows an axial section of a lung from a patient with emphysema. Holes scattered throughout the lung can be seen. These patients have been dubbed "pink puffers."

Type B
A typical presentation would be a man in his 50s with a history of chronic cough with expectoration for several years. This expectoration has gradually increased in severity, being present only in the winter months initially

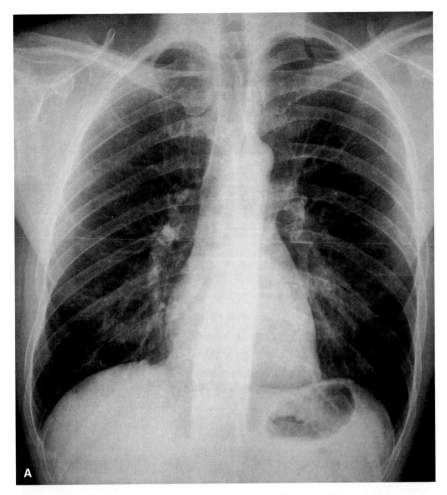

Figure 4.8. Radiographic appearances in the normal lung and in emphysema.
A. Normal lung.

but, more recently, lasting most of the year. Acute exacerbations with frankly purulent sputum have become more common. Shortness of breath on exertion has gradually worsened, with progressively limiting exercise tolerance. The patient is almost invariably a cigarette smoker of many years' duration. This can be quantified as the number of cigarette packs a day multiplied by the number of years of smoking to give the "pack-years."

On examination, the patient has a stocky build with a plethoric complexion and some cyanosis. Auscultation reveals scattered rales (crackles) and rhonchi (whistles). There may be signs of fluid retention with a raised jugular venous pressure and ankle edema. The chest radiograph shows some cardiac

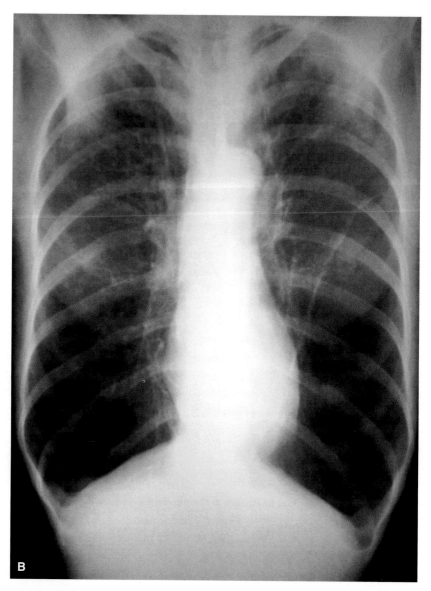

Figure 4.8. (*Continued*) **B.** The pattern of overinflation, with low diaphragms, narrow mediastinum, and increased translucency that is seen in emphysema. The emphysema is particularly prominent in the lower regions of the lung.

enlargement, congested lung fields, and increased markings attributable to old infection. Parallel lines (tram lines) may be seen, probably caused by the thickened walls of inflamed bronchi. At autopsy, chronic inflammatory changes in the bronchi are the rule if the patient had severe bronchitis, but there may be severe emphysema as well. These patients are sometimes called "blue bloaters."

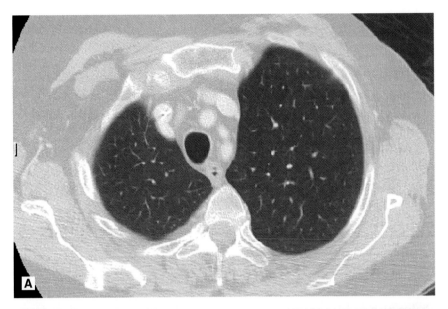

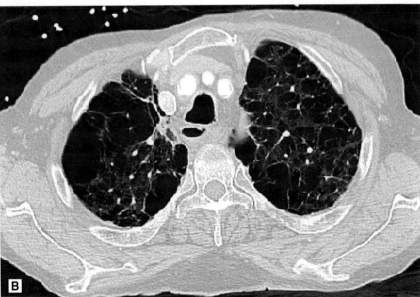

Figure 4.9. A. Appearance of normal lung on CT scan of the chest. **B.** CT scan of the lungs of a patient with emphysema. Holes can be seen scattered throughout the lung.

Some physicians believe that the essential difference between the two types is in the control of breathing. They suggest that the more severe hypoxemia and consequent higher incidence of cor pulmonale in the type B patients can be attributed to a reduced ventilatory drive, especially during sleep.

Features of Type A and Type B Presentations in COPD	
Type A—"Pink Puffer"	**Type B—"Blue Bloater"**
Increasing dyspnea over years	Increasing dyspnea over years
Little or no cough	Frequent cough with sputum
Marked chest overexpansion	Moderate or no increase in chest volume
No cyanosis	Often cyanosis
Quiet breath sounds	Rales and rhonchi
Normal jugular venous pressure	Raised jugular venous pressure
No peripheral edema	Peripheral edema
Arterial P_{O_2} only moderately depressed	P_{O_2} often very low
Arterial P_{CO_2} normal	P_{CO_2} often raised

Pulmonary Function

Most of the features of disordered function in COPD follow from the pathologic features discussed earlier and illustrated in **Figures 4.2 to 4.7.**

Ventilatory Capacity and Mechanics

The forced expiratory volume in 1 second (FEV_1), forced vital capacity (FVC), forced expiratory volume as a percentage of vital capacity (FEV/FVC), forced expiratory flow ($FEF_{25-75\%}$), and maximum expiratory flow at 50% and 75% of exhaled vital capacity ($\dot{V}max_{50\%}$ and $\dot{V}max_{75\%}$) are all reduced. All of these measurements reflect the airway obstruction, whether caused by excessive mucus in the lumen, thickening of the wall by inflammatory changes (see **Figure 4.1A and B**) or by the loss of radial traction (see **Figure 4.1C**). The FVC is reduced because the airways close prematurely during expiration at an abnormally high lung volume, giving an increased residual volume (RV). Again, all three mechanisms of **Figure 4.1** may be contributing factors.

Examination of the spirogram shows that the flow rate over most of the forced expiration is greatly reduced and the *expiratory time* is much increased. Indeed, some physicians regard this prolonged time as a useful simple bedside index of obstruction. Often, the maneuver is terminated by breathlessness when the patient is still exhaling. The low flow rate over most of the forced expiration partly reflects the reduced elastic recoil of the emphysematous lung, which generates the pressure responsible for flow under these conditions of dynamic compression (see Figure 1.6). Typically, the FEV_1 may be reduced to less than 0.8 liters in severe disease, whereas healthy young individuals may have values at or above 4 liters depending on their age, height, and gender (see Appendix A).

In some patients, the FEV_1, FVC, and FEV/FVC may increase significantly after the administration of a bronchodilator aerosol (e.g., 0.5% albuterol by nebulizer for 3 minutes), although the airflow obstruction is incompletely reversible. Significant response to bronchodilators over a period of weeks suggests asthma, and this disease may overlap with chronic bronchitis (asthmatic bronchitis).

The expiratory flow–volume curve is grossly abnormal in severe disease. Figure 1.8 shows that after a brief interval of moderately high flow, flow is strikingly reduced as the airways collapse, and flow limitation by dynamic compression occurs. The graphed curve often has a scooped-out appearance. Flow is greatly reduced in relation to lung volume and ceases at a high lung volume because of premature airway closure (see Figure 1.5B). However, the inspiratory flow–volume curve may be normal or nearly so (see Figure 1.9) as the airways are tethered open by radial traction exerted by the surrounding alveolar walls during inhalation.

The total lung capacity (TLC), functional residual capacity (FRC), and RV are all typically increased in emphysema. Often, the RV/TLC may exceed 40% (less than 30% in young healthy patients). There is often a striking discrepancy between the FRC determined by the body plethysmograph and by the gas dilution techniques (helium equilibration), the former being higher by 1 liter or more. This may be caused by regions of uncommunicating lung behind grossly distorted airways. However, the disparity more often reflects the slow equilibration process in poorly ventilated areas. These static lung volumes are also often abnormal in patients with chronic bronchitis, although the increases in volume are generally less marked.

Elastic recoil of the lung is reduced in emphysema (see Figure 3.1), the pressure–volume curve being displaced up and to the left. This change reflects the disorganization and loss of elastic tissue as a result of the destruction of alveolar walls. The transpulmonary pressure at TLC is low. In uncomplicated chronic bronchitis in the absence of emphysema, the pressure–volume curve may be nearly normal because the parenchyma is little affected.

Airway resistance (related to lung volume) is increased in COPD. All the factors shown in Figure 4.1 may be responsible. However, it is possible to distinguish between an increased resistance caused by intrinsic narrowing of the airway or debris in the lumen (Figure 4.1A and B) and the loss of elastic recoil and radial traction (Figure 4.1C). This can be done by relating resistance to the static elastic recoil.

Figure 4.10 shows airway conductance (reciprocal of resistance) plotted against static transpulmonary pressure in a series of 10 healthy patients, 10 patients with emphysema (without bronchitis), and 10 asthmatics. The measurements were made during a quiet, unforced expiration. Note that the relationship between conductance and transpulmonary pressure for the patients with emphysema was almost normal. In other words, we can ascribe their reduced ventilatory capacity almost entirely to the effects of the smaller elastic recoil pressure of the lung. This not only reduces the effective driving pressure during

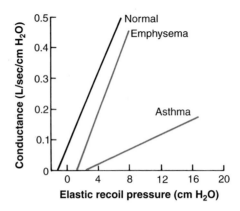

Figure 4.10. Relationships between airway conductance and elastic recoil pressure in obstructive pulmonary disease. Note that the line for emphysema lies close to the normal line. It is evident that any increase in airway resistance is chiefly caused by the smaller elastic recoil of the lung. By contrast, in asthma, the line is markedly abnormal due to the intrinsic narrowing of the airways. (From Colebatch HJH, Finucane KE, Smith MM. Pulmonary conductance and elastic recoil relationships in asthma and emphysema. *J Appl Physiol* 1973;34:143–153.)

a forced expiration but also allows the airways to collapse more easily because of the loss of radial traction. The small displacement of the emphysematous line to the right probably reflects the distortion and loss of airways in this disease.

By contrast, the line for the asthmatics shows that the airway conductance was greatly reduced at a given recoil pressure. Thus, the higher resistance in these patients can be ascribed to intrinsic narrowing of the airways caused by contraction of smooth muscle and inflammatory changes in the airways. After inhalation of a bronchodilator drug, isoproterenol, the asthmatic line moved toward the normal position (not shown in Figure 4.10). Comparable data are not available for a group of patients with chronic bronchitis without emphysema because it is virtually impossible to select such a group during life. However, Figure 4.10 clarifies the behavior of different types of airway obstruction.

Gas Exchange

Ventilation–perfusion inequality is inevitable in COPD and leads to hypoxemia with or without CO_2 retention. Typically, the type A patient has only moderate hypoxemia (P_{O_2} often in the high 60s or 70s), and the arterial P_{CO_2} is normal. By contrast, the type B patient often has severe hypoxemia (P_{O_2} often in the 50s or 40s) with an increased P_{CO_2}, especially in advanced disease.

The alveolar–arterial difference for P_{O_2} is always increased, especially in patients with severe bronchitis. An analysis based on the concept of the ideal point (see Figure 2.7) reveals increases in both physiologic dead space and physiologic shunt. The dead space is particularly increased in emphysema, whereas high values for physiologic shunt are especially common in bronchitis.

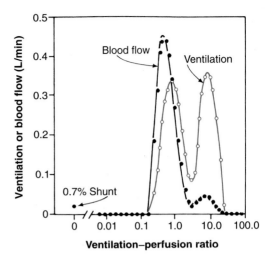

Figure 4.11. Distribution of ventilation–perfusion ratios in a patient with type A COPD. Note the large amount of ventilation to units with high ventilation–perfusion ratios (physiologic dead space). (From Wagner PD, Dantzker DR, Dueck R, et al. Ventilation–perfusion inequality in chronic pulmonary disease. *J Clin Invest* 1977;59:203–206.)

The reasons for these differences are clarified by the results obtained with the inert gas elimination technique. First, review Figure 2.8, which shows a typical pattern in a normal subject. By contrast, **Figure 4.11** shows a typical distribution in a patient with advanced type A disease. This 76-year-old man had a history of increasing dyspnea over several years. The chest radiograph showed hyperinflation with attenuated small pulmonary vessels. The arterial P_{O_2} and P_{CO_2} were 68 and 39 mm Hg, respectively.

The distribution shows that a large amount of ventilation went to lung units with high ventilation–perfusion ratios ($\dot{V}_A / \dot{Q}$) (compare Figure 2.8). This would be shown as physiologic dead space in the ideal point analysis, and the excessive ventilation is largely wasted from the point of view of gas exchange. By contrast, there is little blood flow to units with an abnormally low $\dot{V}_A / \dot{Q}$. This explains the relatively mild degree of hypoxemia in the patient and the fact that the calculated physiologic shunt was only slightly increased.

These findings can be contrasted with those shown in **Figure 4.12**, which shows the distribution in a 47-year-old man with advanced chronic bronchitis and type B disease. He was a heavy smoker and had had a productive cough for many years. The arterial P_{O_2} and P_{CO_2} were 47 and 50 mm Hg, respectively. Note that there was some increase in ventilation to high $\dot{V}_A / \dot{Q}$ units (physiologic dead space). However, the distribution chiefly shows large amounts of blood flow to low $\dot{V}_A / \dot{Q}$ units (physiologic shunt), accounting for his severe hypoxemia. It is remarkable that there was no blood flow to unventilated alveoli (true shunt). Indeed, true shunts of more than a few percent are uncommon in COPD. Note that although the patterns shown in Figures 4.11 and 4.12 are typical, considerable variation is seen in patients with COPD.

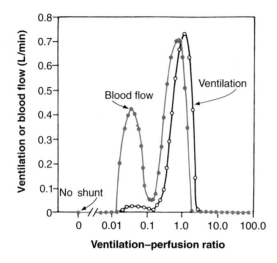

Figure 4.12. Distribution of ventilation–perfusion ratios in a patient with type B COPD. There is a large amount of blood flow to units with low ventilation–perfusion ratios (physiologic shunt). (From Wagner PD, Dantzker DR, Dueck R, et al. Ventilation–perfusion inequality in chronic pulmonary disease. *J Clin Invest* 1977;59:203–206.)

On exercise, the arterial P_{O_2} may fall or rise depending on the response of the ventilation and the cardiac output and the changes in the distribution of ventilation and blood flow. In some patients at least, the main factor in the fall of P_{O_2} is the limited cardiac output, which, in the presence of ventilation–perfusion inequality, exaggerates any hypoxemia. Patients with CO_2 retention often show higher P_{CO_2} values on exercise because of their limited ventilatory response.

The reasons for the ventilation–perfusion inequality are clear when we consider the disorganization of the lung architecture in emphysema (Figures 4.2 and 4.3) and the abnormalities in airways in chronic bronchitis (Figure 4.6). There is ample evidence of uneven ventilation as determined by the single-breath nitrogen washout (see Figure 1.10). In addition, topographic measurements with radioactive materials show regional inequality of both ventilation and blood flow. The blood flow inequality is largely caused by the destruction of portions of the capillary bed.

The deleterious effects of airway obstruction on gas exchange are reduced by collateral ventilation that occurs in these patients. Communicating channels normally exist between adjacent alveoli and between neighboring small airways, and there have been many experimental demonstrations of these. The fact that there is so little blood flow to unventilated units in these patients (Figures 4.11 and 4.12) emphasizes the effectiveness of collateral ventilation because some airways must presumably be completely obstructed, especially in severe bronchitis (see Figure 1.12).

Another factor that reduces the amount of ventilation–perfusion inequality is hypoxic vasoconstriction. (See *West's Respiratory Physiology: The Essentials.* 10th ed. p. 52.) This local response to a low alveolar P_{O_2} reduces the blood flow to poorly ventilated and unventilated regions, minimizing the arterial hypoxemia. When patients with COPD are given bronchodilators, for example, albuterol, they sometimes develop a slight fall in arterial P_{O_2}. This is probably caused by the vasodilator action of these β-adrenergic drugs, increasing the blood flow to poorly ventilated areas. This finding is more marked in asthma (see Figures 4.17 and 4.18).

The arterial P_{CO_2} is often normal in patients with mild to moderate COPD despite their ventilation–perfusion inequality. Any tendency for the arterial P_{CO_2} to rise stimulates the chemoreceptors, thus increasing ventilation to the alveoli (see Figure 2.9). As disease becomes more severe, the arterial P_{CO_2} may rise. This is particularly likely to occur in type B patients. The increased work of breathing is an important factor, but there is also evidence that the sensitivity of the respiratory center to CO_2 is reduced in some of these patients.

If the arterial P_{CO_2} rises, the pH tends to fall, resulting in respiratory acidosis. In some patients, the P_{CO_2} rises so slowly that the kidney is able to compensate adequately by retaining bicarbonate, and the pH remains almost constant (compensated respiratory acidosis). The P_{CO_2} may rise more suddenly during COPD exacerbations or acute chest infections, leading to acute respiratory acidosis (see Chapter 8, Respiratory Failure).

Additional information about gas exchange in these patients can be obtained by measuring the diffusing capacity (transfer factor) for carbon monoxide (see Figure 2.11). The diffusing capacity as measured by the single-breath method is particularly likely to be reduced in patients with severe emphysema. By contrast, patients with chronic bronchitis but little parenchymal destruction may have normal values.

Pulmonary Circulation

The pulmonary artery pressure frequently rises in patients with COPD as their disease progresses. Several factors are responsible. In emphysema, large portions of the capillary bed are destroyed, thus increasing vascular resistance. Hypoxic vasoconstriction also raises the pulmonary arterial pressure, and often, an exacerbation of chest infection causes an additional transient increase as the alveolar hypoxia worsens. Acidosis may exaggerate the hypoxic vasoconstriction. In advanced disease, histologic changes in the walls of the small arteries occur. Finally, these patients often develop polycythemia as a response to the hypoxemia, thus increasing blood viscosity. This occurs most commonly in patients with severe bronchitis, who tend to have the lowest arterial P_{O_2}.

Fluid retention with dependent edema and engorged neck veins may occur, especially in type B patients. The right heart often enlarges with characteristic radiologic and electrocardiographic appearances. The term "cor pulmonale" is given to this condition, but whether it should be regarded as right heart failure is disputed. The output of the heart is normally increased because it is operating high on the Starling curve, and the output can rise further on exercise.

Control of Ventilation

As indicated previously, some patients with COPD, particularly those with severe chronic bronchitis, develop CO_2 retention because they do not sufficiently increase the ventilation to their alveoli. The reasons why some patients behave in this way and some do not are not completely understood. One factor is the increased work of breathing as a result of the high airway resistance. As a consequence, the O_2 cost of breathing may be enormous **(Figure 4.13)**. Normal subjects have an abnormally small ventilatory response to inhaled CO_2 if they are asked to breathe through a high resistance. Thus, a patient with a severely limited O_2 consumption may be willing to forgo a normal arterial P_{CO_2} to obtain the advantage of a reduced work of breathing and a correspondingly reduced O_2 cost. However, the correlation between airway resistance and arterial P_{CO_2} is sufficiently poor that some other factor must be involved.

Measurements of the ventilatory response to inhaled CO_2 show that there are significant differences among normal subjects. These differences are partly caused by genetic factors. Some patients have a reduced respiratory center output in response to inhaled CO_2, many have a mechanical obstruction to ventilation, and some patients have both. Thus, it is possible that the ventilatory response of a patient in the face of severe ventilation–perfusion inequality and increased work of breathing is predetermined to some extent by these factors.

Changes in Early Disease

So far, we have been concerned mainly with pulmonary function in patients with well-established disease. However, relatively little can be done to reverse the disease process in this group, and the treatment is limited chiefly to symptom relief with bronchodilators, prevention and control of infection, and rehabilitative programs. There is a great deal of interest in identifying patients with early disease in the hope that the changes can be arrested or

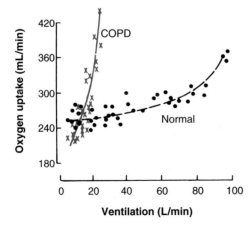

Figure 4.13. Oxygen uptake during voluntary hyperventilation in patients with COPD. Note the high values compared with those of the normal subjects. (From Cherniack RM, Cherniack L, Naimark A. *Respiration in Health and Disease.* 2nd ed. Philadelphia, PA: WB Saunders, 1972.)

reversed by elimination of smoking or other risk factors such as exposuɪ pollution.

It was emphasized in Chapter 1 that because relatively little of the airw ɹy resistance resides in small airways (less than 2 mm wide), pathophysiologic changes there may go unnoticed by the usual function tests. There is some evidence that the earliest changes in COPD occur in these small airways. Interest has focused on whether changes in FEV_1, $FEF_{25-75\%}$, $\dot{V} max_{50\%}$, $\dot{V} max_{75\%}$, and closing volume can be used to identify early disease but their practical value for clinical purposes remains uncertain.

Treatment of Patients with COPD

Smoking cessation is the most critical step for most patients as this is the one intervention that can slow the rate of decline in lung function over time. Exposure to occupational and atmospheric pollution should also be reduced as far as possible. Bronchodilator therapy, including β-agonists and anticholinergics, is the mainstay of therapy for all COPD patients, with the intensity of use varying depending on the severity of the patient's airflow obstruction, functional limitation, and frequency of exacerbations. Inhaled corticosteroids are also used in many patients but are generally reserved for those with more severe disease and/or frequent exacerbations, while the macrolide antibiotic, azithromycin, is now being used on a chronic basis in patients who suffer from frequent exacerbations. Pulmonary rehabilitation can be prescribed to patients with stable disease of any severity and has been shown to quality of life and exercise capacity. Administration of continuous supplemental oxygen to patients with sufficient degrees of chronic hypoxemia is associated with improved survival in such patients. One benefit of this intervention is an increase in the average alveolar P_{O_2}, which lessens hypoxic pulmonary vasoconstriction and partially alleviates the pulmonary hypertension that can occur in severe cases and worsen prognosis.

Lung Volume Reduction Surgery

Surgery to reduce the volume of the overexpanded lung can be valuable in selected cases. The physiologic basis is that reducing the volume increases the radial traction on the airways and therefore helps to limit dynamic compression. In addition, the inspiratory muscles, particularly the diaphragm, are shortened with consequent improvement in their mechanical efficiency. Initially, the emphasis was on resecting bullae, but now, good results can be obtained in patients with more diffuse emphysema. The aim is to remove emphysematous and avascular areas and to preserve the nearly normal regions. Criteria for surgery usually include an FEV_1 of less than 45% predicted, lung volume measurements consistent with air-trapping and hyperinflation, upper lobe predominant emphysema demonstrated by CT scan, and low exercise capacity following a pulmonary rehabilitation program. In properly selected patients, LVRS is associated with improvements in spirometry, lung volumes, quality of life, and dyspnea and, in a small set of patients, improved survival.

ASTHMA

This disease is characterized by increased responsiveness of the airways to various stimuli and is manifested by inflammation and widespread narrowing of the airways that changes in severity, either spontaneously or as a result of treatment.

Pathology

The airways have hypertrophied smooth muscle that contracts during an attack, causing bronchoconstriction **(Figure 4.1B)**. In addition, there is hypertrophy of mucous glands, edema of the bronchial wall, and extensive infiltration by eosinophils and lymphocytes **(Figure 4.15)**. The mucus is increased and is also abnormal; it is thick, tenacious, and slow moving. In severe cases, many airways are occluded by mucous plugs, some of which may be coughed up in the sputum. The sputum typically is scant and white. Subepithelial fibrosis is common in patients with chronic asthma and is part of the process called remodeling. In uncomplicated asthma, there is no destruction of alveolar walls, and there are no copious purulent bronchial secretions. Occasionally, the abundance of eosinophils in the sputum gives a purulent appearance, which may be wrongly ascribed to infection.

Pathogenesis

Two features that appear to be common to all asthmatics are airway hyper-responsiveness and airway inflammation. Research suggests that the hyper-responsiveness is a consequence of the inflammation, and some investigators believe that airway inflammation is responsible for all the associated features

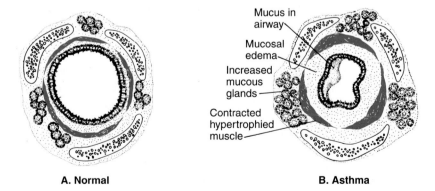

Mucus in airway
Mucosal edema
Increased mucous glands
Contracted hypertrophied muscle

A. Normal   **B. Asthma**

Figure 4.14. Bronchial wall in asthma (diagrammatic). Compared to the normal airway **(A)**, the bronchial wall in asthma **(B)** demonstrates contracted smooth muscle, edema, mucous gland hypertrophy, and secretions in the lumen.

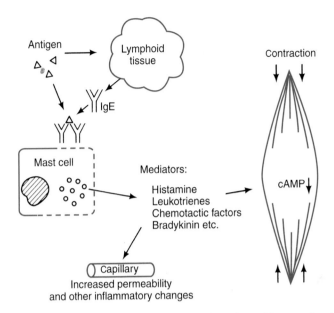

Figure 4.15. **Some pathogenic changes in allergic asthma.** (See text for details.)

of asthma, including the increased airway responsiveness, airway edema, hypersecretion of mucus, and inflammatory cell infiltration. However, a fundamental abnormality of airway smooth muscle or regulation of airway tone is possible in some patients.

Epidemiologic studies indicate that asthma begins in childhood in the majority of cases and that an allergic diathesis often plays an important role. However, environmental factors appear to be important and may be responsible for the increase in the prevalence and severity of asthma over the last 20 to 40 years in modernized, affluent western countries. Frequent exposure to typical childhood infections and environments favoring fecal contamination are associated with a lower incidence of asthma. These observations and others have led to the "hygiene hypothesis," which suggests that children in a critical stage of development of the immune response who are not frequently exposed to typical childhood infectious agents may more frequently develop an allergic diathesis and asthma. Other hypotheses have also been proposed to explain the increases in prevalence including obesity, poor physical fitness, and exposure to pollutants.

The trigger for the development of airway inflammation cannot always be identified. It is well recognized in some instances, as in the case for some antigens in persons with allergic asthma **(Figure 4.15)**. However, in other types of asthma, such as exercise-induced asthma or asthma following a viral respiratory tract infection, the trigger is not recognized. Atmospheric pollutants, especially submicronic particles in automobile exhaust gases, may also play a role.

A single inflammatory cell type or inflammatory mediator does not appear to be responsible for all manifestations of asthma. Eosinophils, mast cells, neutrophils, macrophages, and basophils have all been implicated. There is also evidence that noninflammatory cells, including airway epithelial cells and neural cells, especially those of peptidergic nerves, contribute to the inflammation. Some investigators believe that eosinophils play a central effector role in most cases of asthma. There is also evidence that lympho-cytes, especially T cells, are implicated, both because they respond to spe-cific antigens and because they have a role as a modulator of inflammatory cell function.

Many inflammatory mediators have been identified in asthma. Cytokines are probably important, particularly those associated with Th-2, helper T-cell activation. These cytokines include interleukin-3, IL-4, IL-5, and IL-13. It is believed that these cytokines are at least partly responsible for modulating inflammatory and immune cell function and for supporting the inflammatory response in the airway. Other inflammatory mediators that probably play a role, particularly in acute bronchoconstriction, include arachidonic acid metabo-lites, such as leukotrienes and prostaglandins, platelet-activating factor (PAF), neuropeptides, reactive oxygen species, kinins, histamine, and adenosine.

Asthma also has a genetic component. Population studies show that it is a complex genetic disorder with both environmental and genetic compo-nents. The latter is not a single gene trait but is polygenic. Associations of asthma with a variety of chromosomal loci through linkage analysis have been demonstrated.

Clinical Features

Asthma commonly begins in children but may occur at any age. The patient may have a previous history to suggest atopy, including allergic rhinitis, eczema, or urticaria, and may relate asthmatic attacks to a specific allergen, for example, ragweed or cats. Such a patient is said to have allergic asthma. Many such patients have an increased total serum IgE, increased specific IgE, and peripheral blood eosinophils. If there is no general history of allergy and no external allergen can be identified, the term "nonallergic asthma" is used.

In all asthmatics, there is general hyperreactivity of the airways, with the result that nonspecific irritants, such as smoke, cold air, and exercise, cause symptoms. The hyperreactivity (or hyperresponsiveness) of the airways can be tested by exposing the patient to increasing inhaled concentrations of methacholine or histamine and measuring the FEV_1 (or airway resistance). The concentration that results in a 20% fall in FEV_1 is known as the PC_{20} (provocative concentration 20). This can also be tested by measuring spirom-etry before and after specially designed exercise protocols and demonstrating a decrease in FEV_1 in the postexercise period.

Exacerbations, often referred to as "asthma attacks," may follow changes in air quality, viral infections, or exercise, especially in a cold environment, but can also occur without obvious triggers. Aspirin ingestion is a cause in some individuals because of inhibition of the cyclooxygenase pathway. This may have a genetic component. During an attack, the patient may be extremely dyspneic, orthopneic, and anxious and complain of chest tightness. The accessory muscles of respiration are active. The lungs are hyperinflated, and musical rhonchi are heard in all areas. The pulse is rapid, and pulsus paradoxus may be present (marked fall in systolic and pulse pressure during inspiration). The sputum is scant and viscid. The chest radiograph reveals hyperinflation but is otherwise normal. *Status asthmaticus* refers to an attack that continues for hours or even days without remission despite bronchodilator and corticosteroid therapy. There are often signs of exhaustion, dehydration, and marked tachycardia. The chest may become ominously silent, and vigorous treatment is urgently required.

Depending on the severity of their disease, some patients lack symptoms and have a normal exam and spirometry between exacerbations. Other patients, however, remain symptomatic even when not in an exacerbation and require daily medications for disease control.

Bronchoactive Drugs

Drugs that reverse or prevent bronchoconstriction play a major role in the treatment of patients with asthma.

β-Adrenergic Agonists

β-Adrenergic receptors are of two types: β_1 receptors exist in the heart and elsewhere, and their stimulation increases heart rate and the force of contraction of cardiac muscle. Stimulation of β_2 receptors relaxes smooth muscle in the bronchi, blood vessels, and uterus. Partially or completely β_2-selective adrenergic agonists have now completely replaced nonselective agonists, with the most commonly used agents being albuterol and levalbuterol. These agents have an intermediate duration of action. Long-acting agents, such as formoterol and salmeterol, are also available for daily use but should always be used in combination with inhaled corticosteroids. All these drugs bind to β_2 receptors in the lung and directly relax airway smooth muscle by increasing the activity of adenyl cyclase. This in turn raises the concentration of intracellular cAMP, which is reduced in an asthma attack (Figure 4.15). They also have effects on airway edema and airway inflammation. Their anti-inflammatory effects are mediated by direct inhibition of inflammatory cell function via binding to β_2 receptors on the cell surface. There is some polymorphism in these receptors that affects the responses.

These drugs are delivered by aerosol, preferably using a metered-dose inhaler or a nebulizer. Frequent administration during an asthma attack can be associated with tachyphylaxis. This issue is not generally seen, however, with chronic administration in stable patients.

Inhaled Corticosteroids

Corticosteroids appear to have two separate functions: they inhibit the inflammatory/immune response, and they enhance β receptor expression or function. Because asthma is an inherently inflammatory disorder, inhaled corticosteroids are now the primary controller medication (i.e., routine daily use) in all patients with persistent disease of any severity. This is in contrast to COPD, where inhaled corticosteroids are reserved for those with more severe disease. Current guidelines recommend inhaled corticosteroids for patients with symptoms more than twice a week, inhaled β-agonist use more than twice a week or frequent nighttime awakenings due to asthma symptoms. A wide variety of inhaled corticosteroids are now available and, when used as directed, result in minimal systemic absorption of corticosteroid with almost no serious side effects. In many cases, patients use combination inhalers that deliver both a corticosteroid and a β_2-agonist.

Bronchoactive Drugs for Asthma

β-Adrenergic Agonists
Selective β_2 types are now exclusively used.

Long-acting forms are useful in chronic disease management but should only be used in conjunction with inhaled corticosteroids.

Short-acting forms are reserved for rescue.

Inhaled Corticosteroids
These are given by aerosol and are often indicated except in the mildest cases of asthma.

Auxiliary Drugs
Antileukotrienes, methylxanthine, and cromolyn may be useful adjuncts.

Anticholinergics

While anticholinergics are used extensively in management of patients with COPD, they are generally not part of the treatment regimen in the majority of asthma patients. This is despite some evidence that the parasympathetic system plays a role in asthma pathophysiology. Some recent evidence suggests the long-acting anticholinergic tiotropium may have benefit in patients with persistent symptoms despite intensive therapy with inhaled corticosteroids and β_2-agonists, but this is not presently standard practice.

Cromolyn and Nedocromil

Although their precise mechanism of action remains unclear, these two drugs are thought to prevent bronchoconstriction by stabilizing mast cells **(Figure 4.15)** and other broad ranging effects. Their use is generally limited to prophylaxis in situations known to provoke symptoms such as prior to exercise in cold, dry conditions, or visiting an environment with a known trigger for the particular patient such as a home with a cat.

Methylxanthines
Methylxanthines, including theophylline and aminophylline, inhibit phosphodiesterases in bronchial smooth muscle, leading to bronchodilation. While used more extensively in the past, they are used little in current practice because of modest anti-inflammatory and bronchodilatory activity relative to corticosteroids and β_2-agonists, risk for toxicity, and the need for monitoring serum concentrations on a regular basis.

Leukotriene-Modifying Drugs
Because leukotrienes C4, D4, and E4 have increasingly been recognized to mediate part of the allergic response in asthma, leukotriene receptor antagonists (e.g., montelukast, zafirlukast) and 5-lipoxygenase inhibitors (e.g., zileuton) are now used in some individuals. In well-selected patients with mild to moderate disease, they can be used in lieu of inhaled corticosteroids, while in more severe forms of disease, they may provide benefit when added to existing treatment with inhaled corticosteroids. They may be of particular use to patients whose asthma is exacerbated by aspirin and other nonsteroidal anti-inflammatory drugs.

Anti-IgE Therapy
A monoclonal antibody to IgE, omalizumab, is now available for use in patients with moderate to severe asthma who are inadequately controlled with high doses of inhaled glucocorticoids and have elevated serum IgE levels and evidence of allergen sensitization. Use has been limited by difficulties predicting which patients respond to therapy, the very high cost and the risk of hypersensitivity reactions including anaphylaxis.

Pulmonary Function

As was the case with chronic bronchitis and emphysema, the changes in lung function generally follow clearly from the pathology of asthma.

Ventilatory Capacity and Mechanics
During an attack, all indices of expiratory flow rate are reduced significantly, including the FEV_1, FEV/FVC, $FEF_{25-75\%}$, $\dot{V}max_{50\%}$, and $\dot{V}max_{75\%}$. The FVC is also usually reduced because airways close prematurely toward the end of a full expiration. Between attacks, some impairment of ventilatory capacity can usually be demonstrated, although the patient may report no symptoms and have a normal physical exam.

The response of these indices to bronchodilator drugs is of great importance in asthma **(Figure 4.16)**. They may be tested by administering 0.5% albuterol by aerosol for 2 minutes or several puffs from a metered-dose

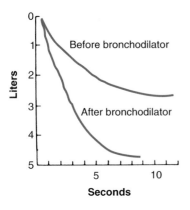

Figure 4.16. **Examples of forced expirations before and after bronchodilator therapy in a patient with bronchial asthma.** Note the striking increase in flow rate and vital capacity. (From Bates DV, Macklem PT, Christie RV. *Respiratory Function in Disease.* 2nd ed. Philadelphia, PA: WB Saunders, 1971.)

inhaler. Typically, all indices increase substantially when a bronchodilator is administered to a patient during an attack, and the change is a valuable measure of the responsiveness of the airways. The extent of the increase varies according to the severity of the disease. In status asthmaticus, little change may be seen because the bronchi have become unresponsive (although pulmonary function tests are rarely measured during such acute presentations). Again, patients in remission may show only minor improvement following bronchodilator administration, although generally there is some.

There is some evidence that the relative change in FEV_1 and FVC after bronchodilator therapy indicates whether the bronchospasm has been completely relieved. During an asthma attack, both the FEV_1 and FVC tend to increase by the same fraction, with the result that the FEV/FVC remains low and almost constant. However, when the tone of the airway muscle is nearly normal, the FEV_1 responds more than the FVC, and the FEV/FVC approaches the normal value of approximately 75%.

The flow–volume curve in asthma has the typical obstructive pattern, although it may not exhibit the scooped-out appearance seen in emphysema (see Figure 1.8). After a bronchodilator, flows are higher at all lung volumes, and the whole curve may shift as the TLC and RV are reduced.

Static lung volumes are increased, and remarkably high values for FRC and TLC during asthma attacks have been reported. The increased RV is caused by premature airway closure during a full expiration as a result of the increased smooth muscle tone, edema and inflammation of the airway walls, and abnormal secretions. The cause of the increased FRC and TLC is not fully understood. However, there is some loss of elastic recoil, and the pressure–volume curve is shifted upward and to the left (see Figure 3.1). This tends to return toward normal after a bronchodilator has been given. There is some evidence that changes in the surface tension of the alveolar lining layer may be responsible for the altered elastic properties. The rise in lung volume tends to decrease resistance of the airways by increasing their radial traction. The FRC measured by helium dilution is usually considerably below that found with the body plethysmograph, reflecting the presence of occluded airways or the delayed equilibration of poorly ventilated areas.

Airway resistance as measured in the body plethysmograph is raised, and it falls after a bronchodilator. It is likely that the broncho-spasm affects airways of all sizes, and the relationship between airway conductance and elastic recoil pressure is significantly abnormal (Figure 4.10). Narrowing of the large- and medium-sized bronchi can be seen directly at bronchoscopy.

Gas Exchange

Arterial hypoxemia is common in asthma and is caused by ventilation–perfusion $(\dot{V}_A/\dot{Q})$ inequality. There is ample evidence of uneven ventilation, and measurements with radioactive gases show regions of reduced ventilation. Marked topographical inequality of blood flow is also seen, and typically, different areas show transient reductions at different times. Both physiologic dead space and physiologic shunt are generally abnormally high.

An example of a distribution of ventilation–perfusion ratios in a 47-year-old asthmatic is shown in **Figure 4.17**. This patient had only mild symptoms at the time of the measurement. The distribution is strikingly different from the normal distribution shown in Figure 2.8. Note especially the bimodal distribution with a considerable amount of the total blood flow (approximately 25%) to units with a low $\dot{V}_A/\dot{Q}$ (approximately 0.1). This accounts for the patient's mild hypoxemia, the arterial P_{O_2} being

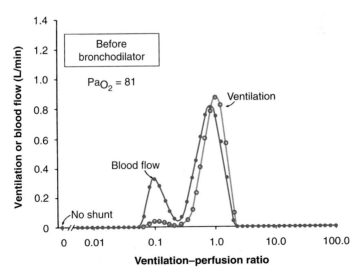

Figure 4.17. Distribution of ventilation–perfusion ratios in a patient with asthma.
Note the bimodal appearance, with approximately 25% of the blood flowing to units with ventilation–perfusion ratios in the region of 0.1.

81 mm Hg. There is no pure shunt (blood flow to unventilated alveoli), a surprising finding in view of the mucous plugging of airways, which is a feature of the disease.

When this patient was given the bronchodilator isoproterenol by aerosol, there was an increase in $FEF_{25-75\%}$ from 3.4 to 4.2 L/sec. Thus, there was some relief of his bronchospasm. The changes in the distribution of ventilation–perfusion ratios are shown in **Figure 4.18**. Note that the blood flow to the low $\dot{V}_A/\dot{Q}$ alveoli increased from approximately 25% to 50% of the flow, resulting in a fall in arterial P_{O_2} from 81 to 70 mm Hg. The mean $\dot{V}_A/\dot{Q}$ of the low mode increased slightly from 0.10 to 0.14, indicating that the ventilation to these units increased slightly more than their blood flow. Again, no shunt was seen.

Many bronchodilators, including isoproterenol, aminophylline, and terbutaline, decrease the arterial P_{O_2} in asthmatics. The mechanism of the increased hypoxemia is apparently relief of vasoconstriction in poorly ventilated areas. This vasoconstriction probably results from the release of mediators, like the bronchoconstriction. The fall in P_{O_2} is accompanied by increases in physiologic shunt and dead space. However, in practice, the favorable effects of the drugs on airway resistance far exceed the disadvantages of the mild additional hypoxemia.

The absence of shunt—that is, blood flow to unventilated lung units—in Figures 4.17 and 4.18 is striking, especially because asthmatics who come to autopsy have mucous plugs in many of their airways. Presumably, the explanation is collateral ventilation that reaches the lung situated behind completely closed bronchioles. This is shown diagrammatically in Figure 1.11. The same mechanism probably exists in the lungs of patients with chronic bronchitis (see, e.g., Figure 4.12).

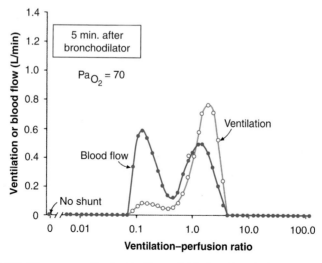

Figure 4.18. The same patient as in Figure 4.16 after the administration of the bronchodilator isoproterenol by aerosol. Note the increase in blood flow to the units with low ventilation–perfusion ratios and the corresponding fall in arterial P_{O_2}.

The arterial P_{CO_2} in patients with asthma is typically normal or low, at least until late in the disease. The P_{CO_2} is prevented from rising by increased ventilation to the alveoli in the face of the ventilation–perfusion inequality (compare Figure 2.9). In many patients, the P_{CO_2} may be in the middle or low 30s during an exacerbation, possibly as a result of stimulation of the peripheral chemoreceptors by the mild hypoxemia or stimulation of intrapulmonary receptors.

In status asthmaticus, the arterial P_{CO_2} may begin to rise and the pH to fall. This is an ominous development that denotes impending respiratory failure and signals the need for urgent and intensive treatment, including possibly mechanical ventilatory support (see Chapter 10). Death can occur in severe asthma exacerbations, often as a result of respiratory failure, because the severity of the disease was not sufficiently appreciated and the patient was initially undertreated.

The diffusing capacity for carbon monoxide is typically normal or high in uncomplicated asthma. If it is reduced, associated emphysema should be suspected. The reason for the increased diffusing capacity is probably the large lung volume. Hyperinflation increases the diffusing capacity in normal subjects, presumably by increasing the area of the blood–gas interface.

LOCALIZED AIRWAY OBSTRUCTION

So far, this chapter has been devoted to generalized airway obstruction, both irreversible, as in emphysema and chronic bronchitis, and reversible, as in asthma. (Some chronic bronchitis may show some reversibility.) Localized obstruction is less common and associated with varying degrees of functional impairment depending on the nature and severity of the obstruction. Obstruction may be within the lumen of the airway, in the wall, or as a result of compression from outside the wall (Figure 4.1).

Tracheal Obstruction

This can be caused by an inhaled foreign body; stenosis after the use of an indwelling tracheostomy tube; intraluminal masses; or compression from extraluminal masses, such as an enlarged thyroid or massive mediastinal lymphadenopathy. There is inspiratory and expiratory stridor, abnormal inspiratory and expiratory flow–volume curves (see Figure 1.9), and no response to bronchodilators. Hypoventilation may result in hypercapnia and hypoxemia (see Figure 2.2).

Bronchial Obstruction

This is often caused by inhalation of a foreign body, such as a peanut or marble. The right lung is more frequently affected than the left because the left main bronchus makes a sharper angle with the trachea than does the right.

Other common causes are bronchial tumors, either malignant or benign, and compression of a bronchus by enlarged surrounding lymph nodes. This last cause particularly affects the right middle lobe bronchus because of its anatomic relationships.

If obstruction is complete, absorption atelectasis occurs because the sum of the partial pressures in mixed venous blood is less than that in alveolar gas. (See *West's Respiratory Physiology: The Essentials.* 10th ed. p. 168.) The collapsed lobe is often visible on the radiograph, and compensatory overinflation of adjacent lung and displacement of a fissure may also be seen. Perfusion of the unventilated lung is reduced because of hypoxic vasoconstriction and also the increased vascular resistance caused by the mechanical effects of the reduced volume on the extra-alveolar vessels and the capillaries. However, the residual blood flow contributes to hypoxemia. The most sensitive test is the alveolar–arterial P_{O_2} difference during 100% O_2 breathing (see Figure 2.6). Infection may follow localized obstruction and lead to lung abscess. If the obstruction is in a segmental or smaller bronchus, atelectasis may not occur because of collateral ventilation (see Figure 1.11). Long-standing unresolved bronchial obstruction can lead to infection and bronchiectasis distal to the obstruction.

KEY CONCEPTS

1. Chronic obstructive pulmonary disease is extremely common and can be very disabling. These patients have emphysema, chronic bronchitis, or a mixture of both.

2. Emphysema is a disease of the lung parenchyma characterized by the breakdown of alveolar walls with loss of lung elastic recoil and dynamic compression of airways.

3. Chronic bronchitis refers to inflammation of the airways with excessive mucus production. The lung parenchyma is normal or nearly so.

4. Asthma is characterized by increased responsiveness of the airways accompanied by inflammation. The airway narrowing typically varies in severity over time.

5. All of these diseases cause marked changes in forced expirations with reductions in the FEV_1, FVC, and FEV/FVC.

6. Asthma can be treated effectively with inhaled corticosteroids and β_2-adrenergic agonists.

7. In addition to smoking cessation, inhaled β_2-adrenergic agonists and anticholinergics are the mainstay of therapy for patients with COPD. Inhaled corticosteroids are usually reserved for severely affected patients.

CLINICAL VIGNETTE

A 26-year-old man comes to the emergency department with worsening dyspnea and chest tightness over a 2-day period. He has had increasing nonproductive cough and states that he feels as if he can't get air into his chest on inhalation. He was diagnosed with asthma several years ago and has been treated with daily inhaled corticosteroids and short-acting β_2-agonist as needed for several years with good improvement. However, following an upper respiratory tract infection that started several days ago, he has taken his β_2-agonist on a more frequent basis for relief of increased symptoms. Today, he has had little relief with the inhaler and decided to seek further help. On examination in the emergency department, his vital signs include temperature 37.0°C, heart rate 110, blood pressure 110/75, respiratory rate 25, and S_pO_2 92% breathing ambient air. His sternocleidomastoid and intercostal muscles are visibly contracting. He has diffuse, musical sounds through his bilateral lung fields and a prolonged expiratory phase. A chest radiograph shows no focal opacities but enlarged rib spaces and flattened diaphragms bilaterally.

Questions
- How would his functional residual capacity and residual volume at present compare to when he is in his normal healthy state?
- Why does he feel as if he can't inhale adequately when asthma is a disease of airflow obstruction on exhalation?
- What is the most likely cause of his hypoxemia?
- If you were to obtain an arterial blood gas, what change would you expect to see in his Pa_{CO_2}?
- What treatment is appropriate at this time?

QUESTIONS

1. Which form of emphysema predominantly affects the apex of the lung?
   A. That caused by α_1-antitrypsin deficiency
   B. Centriacinar emphysema
   C. Panacinar emphysema
   D. Paraseptal emphysema
   E. Unilateral emphysema

2. Patients with COPD with the type A presentation (as opposed to type B) tend to have:
A. more cough productive of sputum.
B. smaller lung volumes.
C. decreased lung elastic recoil.
D. more hypoxemia.
E. greater tendency to develop cor pulmonale.

3. When a bronchodilator is administered to a patient during an asthma attack, which of the following typically decreases?
A. FEV_1
B. FEV/FVC
C. FVC
D. $FEF_{25-75\%}$
E. FRC

4. A 58-year-old man with a 60-pack-year history of smoking comes to the clinic because of worsening dyspnea over a 1-year period. He has no cough. On exam, he is a thin man with scattered musical sounds heard on auscultation and a prolonged expiratory phase. Spirometry performed in clinic shows an FEV_1 45% predicted, FVC 65% predicted, and FEV_1/FVC 0.58. Which of the following would most likely be seen in PA and lateral chest radiographs in this patient?
A. Bilateral hilar lymphadenopathy
B. Decreased size of the retrosternal airspace
C. Decreased vascular markings
D. Diffuse, bilateral lung opacities
E. Reticular opacities at the lung bases

5. A 22-year-old woman presents with episodic dyspnea, chest tightness, and cough. She was seen several months ago for these symptoms at an urgent care clinic and was given an albuterol inhaler, which provided symptomatic relief. She has been using it over five times per week and at least two times per week at night when she awakens with symptoms. Spirometry reveals an FEV_1 65% predicted, FVC 80% predicted, and FEV_1/FVC 0.65. All of these measurements improve significantly following administration of an inhaled bronchodilator. Which of the following medications is indicated for daily use for improved disease control?
A. Anti-IgE therapy
B. Cromolyn
C. Inhaled long-acting anticholinergic
D. Inhaled corticosteroid
E. Inhaled long-acting β_2-agonist

6. A 38-year-old man with only a 5-pack-year history of smoking comes to the pulmonary clinic because of worsening dyspnea on exertion. On exam, he has expiratory wheezes and a long expiratory phase. Pulmonary function testing reveals airflow obstruction without a bronchodilator response, while a plain chest radiograph demonstrates large lung volumes, flat diaphragms, and increased lucency in the bilateral lower lung zones. Which of the following statements is true regarding this patient?
   A. He is not at risk for extrapulmonary disease.
   B. He should be tested for α_1-antitrypsin deficiency.
   C. He is likely a heterozygote for the Z gene.
   D. There is no effective treatment.
   E. Unilateral emphysema is commonly seen in this disease.

7. A 63-year-old woman is evaluated for worsening dyspnea on exertion over an 18-month period. She is a retired teacher with a 30-year history of smoking. Her spirometry reveals an FEV_1 59% predicted, FVC 78% predicted, and FEV_1/FVC ratio 0.62 with no response to inhaled bronchodilators. A chest radiograph demonstrates large lung volumes, a large retrosternal airspace, and flattened diaphragms. Which of the following would most likely be seen on further pulmonary function testing in this patient?
   A. Decreased functional residual capacity
   B. Decreased RV/TLC ratio
   C. Decreased total lung capacity
   D. Increased diffusing capacity for carbon monoxide
   E. Increased residual volume

8. A 16-year-old girl with a history of asthma is brought into the emergency department with chest tightness and wheezing that have not improved despite using her inhaled bronchodilator. On exam, she has an oxygen saturation of 92% breathing ambient air, use of accessory muscles of respiration, and diffuse musical sounds on expiration. An arterial blood gas is drawn and shows a P_{CO_2} 33 mm Hg and P_{O_2} 62 mm Hg. The P_{O_2} improves to 90 mm Hg with administration of 2 L/min of oxygen by nasal cannula. Which of the following is the most likely cause of her hypoxemia?
   A. Diffusion impairment
   B. Hyperventilation
   C. Hypoventilation
   D. Shunt
   E. Ventilation–perfusion mismatch

RESTRICTIVE DISEASES

5

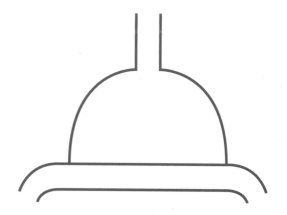

- **Diseases of the Lung Parenchyma**
  Structure of the Alveolar Wall
    Cell Types
    Interstitium
  Diffuse Interstitial Pulmonary Fibrosis
    Pathology
    Pathogenesis
    Clinical Features
    Pulmonary Function
    Treatment and Outcomes
  Other Types of Parenchymal Restrictive Disease
    Sarcoidosis
    Hypersensitivity Pneumonitis
    Interstitial Disease Caused by Drugs, Poisons, and Radiation
    Asbestosis
    Collagen Vascular Diseases
    Lymphangitis Carcinomatosa

- **Diseases of the Pleura**
  Pneumothorax
    Spontaneous Pneumothorax
    Tension Pneumothorax
    Pulmonary Function
  Pleural Effusion
  Pleural Thickening

- **Diseases of the Chest Wall**
  Scoliosis
  Ankylosing Spondylitis

- **Neuromuscular Disorders**

Restrictive diseases are those in which the expansion of the lung is restricted either because of alterations in the lung parenchyma or because of disease of the pleura, the chest wall, or the neuromuscular apparatus. They are characterized by a reduced vital capacity and a small resting lung volume (usually), but the airway resistance (related to lung volume) is not increased. These diseases are therefore different from the obstructive diseases in their pure form, although mixed restrictive and obstructive conditions can occur.

DISEASES OF THE LUNG PARENCHYMA

This term refers to the alveolar tissue of the lung. A brief review of the structure of this tissue is pertinent.

Structure of the Alveolar Wall

Figure 5.1 shows an electron micrograph of a pulmonary capillary in an alveolar wall. The various structures through which oxygen passes on its way from the alveolar gas to the hemoglobin of the red blood cell are the layer of pulmonary surfactant (not shown in this preparation), alveolar epithelium, interstitium, capillary endothelium, plasma, and erythrocyte.

Cell Types
The various cell types have different functions and different responses to injury.

Type 1 Epithelial Cell
This is the chief structural cell of the alveolar wall; its long cytoplasmic extensions pave almost the whole alveolar surface (Figure 5.1). The main function of this cell is mechanical support. It rarely divides and is not very active metabolically. When type 1 cells are injured, they are replaced by type 2 cells, which later transform into type 1 cells.

Type 2 Epithelial Cell
This is a nearly globular cell **(Figure 5.2)** that gives little structural support to the alveolar wall but is metabolically active. The electron micrograph shows the lamellated bodies that contain phospholipids. These are formed in the endoplasmic reticulum, passed through the Golgi apparatus, and eventually extruded into the alveolar space to form surfactant (see *West's Respiratory Physiology: The Essentials*. 10th ed. p. 114). After injury to the alveolar wall, these cells rapidly divide to line the surface and then later transform into type 1 cells. A type 3 cell has also been described, but it is rare and its function is unknown.

Alveolar Macrophage
This scavenger cell roams around the alveolar wall phagocytosing foreign particles and bacteria. The cell contains lysozymes that digest engulfed foreign matter.

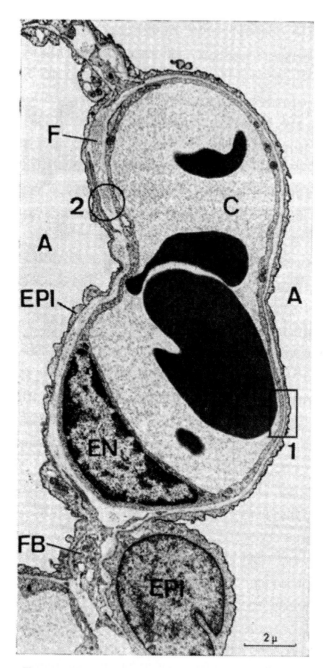

Figure 5.1. Electron micrograph of a portion of an alveolar wall. *(A)* alveolar space; *(EPI)* type I alveolar epithelial cell nucleus and cytoplasm; *(C)* capillary lumen; *(EN)* endothelial cell nucleus; *(FB)* fibroblast; *(F)* collagen fibrils; *(1)* thin region of blood–gas barrier; *(2)* thick region of blood–gas barrier. (From Weibel ER. Morphological basis of alveolar-capillary gas exchange. *Physiolo Res* 1973;53:419–495.)

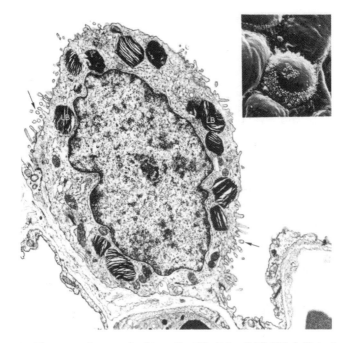

Figure 5.2. Electron micrograph of type 2 epithelial cell (10,000×). Note the lamellated bodies *(LB)*, large nucleus, and microvilli (*arrows*), which are mainly concentrated around the edge of the cell, and cytoplasm rich in organelles. The **inset** at top right is a scanning electron micrograph showing the surface view of a type 2 cell with its characteristic distribution of microvilli (3,400×). (From Weibel ER, Gil J. Structure–function relationships at the alveolar level. In: West JB, ed. *Bioengineering Aspects of the Lung.* New York, NY: Marcel Dekker, 1977.)

Fibroblast

This cell synthesizes collagen and elastin, which are components of the interstitium of the alveolar wall. After various disease insults, large amounts of these materials may be laid down. This results in interstitial fibrosis.

Interstitium

This fills the space between the alveolar epithelium and the capillary endothelium. Figure 5.1 shows that it is thin on one side of the capillary, where it consists only of the fused basement membranes of the epithelial and endothelial layers. On the other side of the capillary, the interstitium is usually wider and includes fibrils of type I collagen. The thick side is chiefly concerned with fluid exchange across the endothelium, whereas the thin side is responsible for most of the gas exchange.

Interstitial tissue is found elsewhere in the lung, notably in the perivascular and peribronchial spaces around the larger blood vessels and airways and in the interlobular septa. The interstitium of the alveolar wall is continuous with that in the perivascular spaces (see Figure 6.1) and is the route by which fluid drains from the capillaries to the lymphatics.

Diffuse Interstitial Pulmonary Fibrosis

The nomenclature of this condition is confusing. Synonyms include idiopathic pulmonary fibrosis, interstitial pneumonia, and cryptogenic fibrosing alveolitis. Some physicians reserve the term "fibrosis" for the late stages of the disease. The changes in pulmonary function are described in detail because they are typical of many of the other conditions alluded to later in this chapter.

Pathology

The principal feature is thickening of the interstitium of the alveolar wall. Initially, there is infiltration with lymphocytes and plasma cells. Later, fibroblasts appear and lay down thick collagen bundles (**Figure 5.3**). These changes may be dispersed irregularly within the lung. In some patients, a cellular

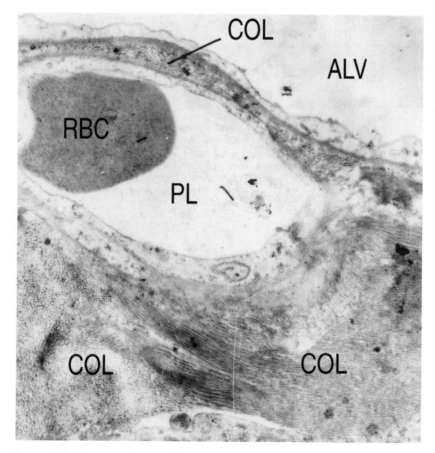

Figure 5.3. Electron micrograph from a patient with diffuse interstitial fibrosis.
Note the thick bundles of collagen. *COL*, collagen; *ALV*, alveolar space; *RBC*, red blood cell; *PL*, plasma. Compare Figure 5.1. (From Gracey DR, Divertie MD, Brown AL Jr. Alveolar–capillary membrane in idiopathic interstitial pulmonary fibrosis. Electron microscopic study of 14 cases. *Am Rev Respir Dis* 1968;98:16–21.)

exudate consisting of macrophages and other mononuclear cells is seen within the alveoli in the early stages of the disease. This is called "desquamation." Eventually, the alveolar architecture is destroyed and the scarring results in multiple air-filled cystic spaces formed by dilated terminal and respiratory bronchioles, so-called honeycomb lung.

Pathogenesis
This is unknown, although in some cases there is evidence of an immunologic reaction.

Clinical Features
The disease is not common and tends to affect adults in the fifth to seventh decades of life. The patient often presents with dyspnea, which is typically more significant on exercise, as well as rapid, shallow breathing. Patients often have an irritating, unproductive cough but lack fevers, hemoptysis, chest pain, and constitutional symptoms.

On examination, mild cyanosis may be seen at rest in severe cases. It typically worsens on exercise. Fine crepitations, often referred to as crackles, are usually heard throughout both lungs, especially toward the end of inspiration. Finger clubbing is common. The chest radiograph (**Figure 5.4**) shows a reticular or reticulonodular pattern, especially at the bases. Patchy shadows near the diaphragm may be caused by basal collapse. Late in the disease, a honeycomb pattern develops, which is best appreciated on a CT scan of the chest; this is caused by multiple airspaces surrounded by thickened tissue (**Figure 5.5**). CT may also show airways that are pulled open by surrounding fibrous tissue, a phenomenon referred to as traction dilatation. The lungs are typically small, and the diaphragms are raised.

Cor pulmonale may develop as a complication of advanced disease. The diseases often progress insidiously and patients typically die from terminal respiratory failure within a few years of diagnosis. Some patients develop acute exacerbations over a period of days to weeks that are associated with a very high risk of mortality.

Pulmonary Function
Ventilatory Capacity and Mechanics
Spirometry typically reveals a restrictive pattern (see Figure 1.2). The FVC is markedly reduced, but the gas is exhaled rapidly so that although the FEV_1 is low, the FEV/FVC is normal or is abnormally high. The almost square shape of the forced expiratory spirogram is in striking contrast to the obstructive pattern (compare Figure 4.16). The $FEF_{25-75\%}$ is normal or high. The flow–volume curve does not show the scooped-out shape of obstructive disease, and the flow rate is often higher than normal when related to absolute lung volume. This is shown in Figure 1.5, where it can be seen that the downslope of the curve for restrictive disease lies above the normal curve.

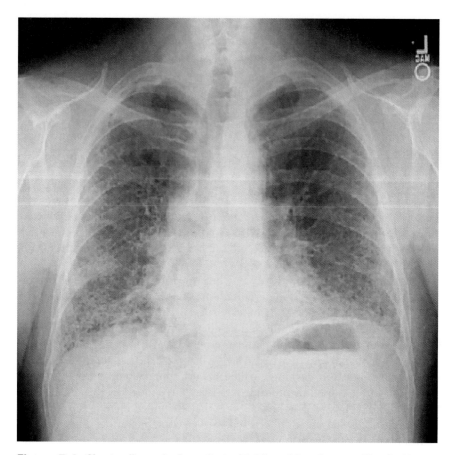

Figure 5.4. Chest radiograph of a patient with idiopathic pulmonary fibrosis. Note the small contracted lung and rib cage and the raised diaphragms. Netlike or "reticular" opacities are present in both lungs, particularly at the lung bases. Compare the normal appearance in Figure 4.8A.

All lung volumes are reduced, including the TLC, FRC, and RV, but the relative proportions are more or less preserved. The pressure–volume curve of the lung is flattened and displaced downward (see Figure 3.1), so that at any given volume, the transpulmonary pressure is abnormally high. The maximum elastic recoil pressure that can be generated at TLC is typically higher than normal.

All these results are consistent with the pathologic appearance of fibrosis of the alveolar walls (Figures 2.5 and 5.3). The fibrous tissue reduces the distensibility of the lung just as a scar on the skin reduces its extensibility. As a result, the lung volumes are small, and abnormally large pressures are required to distend the lung. The airways may not be specifically involved, but they tend to narrow as lung volume is reduced. However, airway resistance at a given lung volume is normal or even decreased because the retractile forces exerted on the airway walls by the surrounding parenchyma are abnormally

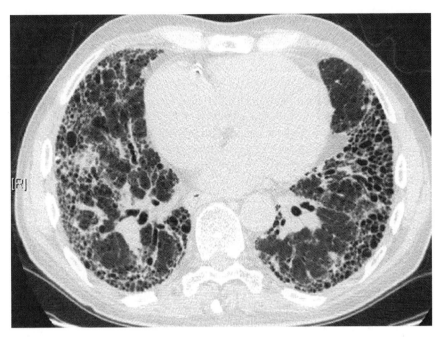

Figure 5.5. Single slice of a chest CT scan of a patient with idiopathic pulmonary fibrosis. Note the extensive septal thickening and the prominent honeycombing, particularly in the periphery of the lungs.

high (**Figure 5.6**). The pathologic correlate of this is the honeycomb appearance caused by the dilated terminal and respiratory bronchioles surrounded by thickened scar tissue.

Gas Exchange

The arterial P_{O_2} and P_{CO_2} are typically reduced, and the pH is normal. The hypoxemia is usually mild at rest until the disease is advanced. However, on

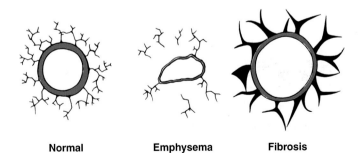

Figure 5.6. Airway caliber in emphysema and interstitial fibrosis. In emphysema, the airways tend to collapse because of the loss of radial traction. By contrast, in fibrosis, radial traction may be excessive, with the result that airway caliber is large when related to lung volume.

exercise, the P_{O_2} often falls dramatically and cyanosis may be evident. In well-established disease, both the physiologic dead space and the physiologic shunt are increased.

The relative contribution of diffusion impairment and ventilation–perfusion ($\dot{V}_A/\dot{Q}$) inequality to the hypoxemia of these patients has long been debated. It is natural to argue that the histologic appearances shown in Figures 2.5 and 5.3 slow the diffusion of oxygen from the alveolar gas to the capillary blood because the thickness of the barrier may be increased manyfold (compare Figure 5.1). In addition, the increasing hypoxemia during exercise is consistent with the mechanism of impaired diffusion because exercise reduces the time spent by the red cells in the pulmonary capillary (Figure 2.4).

However, we now know that impaired diffusion is not the chief cause of the hypoxemia in these conditions. First, the normal lung has enormous reserves of diffusion in that the P_{O_2} of the blood nearly reaches that in alveolar gas early in its transit through the capillary (see Figure 2.4). In addition, these patients have substantial inequality of ventilation and blood flow within the lung. How could they not, with the disorganization of architecture shown in Figures 2.5 and 5.3? The inequalities have been demonstrated by single-breath nitrogen washouts and measurements of topographical function with radioactive gases.

To apportion blame for the hypoxemia between the two possible mechanisms, it is necessary to measure the degree of $\dot{V}_A/\dot{Q}$ inequality and determine how much of the hypoxemia is attributable to this. This has been done by using the multiple inert gas elimination technique in a series of patients with interstitial lung disease. **Figure 5.7** shows that at rest, the hypoxemia could be adequately explained by the degree of $\dot{V}_A/\dot{Q}$ inequality in these patients. However, **Figure 5.8** shows that on exercise, the observed alveolar

Features of Pulmonary Function in Diffuse Interstitial Fibrosis

- Dyspnea with shallow, rapid breathing
- Reductions in all lung volumes
- FEV_1/FVC ratio normal or even increased
- Airway resistance normal or low when related to lung volume
- Reduced lung compliance
- Very negative intrapleural pressure at TLC
- Arterial hypoxemia chiefly due to $\dot{V}_A/\dot{Q}$ inequality
- Diffusion impairment possibly contributing to the hypoxemia during exercise
- Normal or low arterial P_{CO_2}
- Reduced diffusing capacity for carbon monoxide
- Increased pulmonary vascular resistance

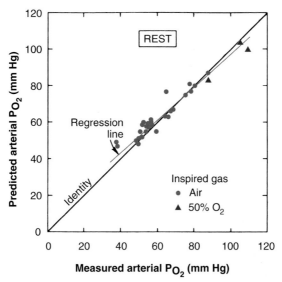

Figure 5.7. **Study of the mechanism of hypoxemia in a series of patients with interstitial lung disease.** This figure shows that the arterial P_{O_2} predicted from the pattern of $\dot{V}_A/\dot{Q}$ inequality agreed well with the measured arterial P_{O_2}. Thus, at rest, all of the hypoxemia could be explained by the uneven ventilation and blood flow.

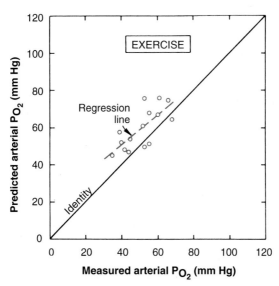

Figure 5.8. **Results obtained on exercise in the same patients as shown in Figure 5.7.** Under these conditions, the measured arterial P_{O_2} was below that predicted from the pattern of $\dot{V}_A/\dot{Q}$ inequality. This indicates an additional mechanism for hypoxemia, presumably diffusion impairment.

P_{O_2} was generally below the value predicted from the measured amount of $\dot{V}_A/\dot{Q}$ inequality, and thus, an additional cause of hypoxemia must have been present. Most likely, this was diffusion impairment in these patients. However, hypoxemia caused by diffusion impairment was evident only on exercise, and even then, it accounted for only about one-third of the alveolar–arterial difference for P_{O_2}.

The low arterial P_{CO_2} in these patients (typically in the low to middle 30s) occurs despite the evident $\dot{V}_A/\dot{Q}$ inequality and is caused by increased ventilation to the alveoli (compare Figure 2.9). The cause of the increased ventilation is uncertain. There is some evidence that the control of ventilation is abnormal because of the stimulation of receptors within the lung (see later text). Stimulation of the peripheral chemoreceptors by the arterial hypoxemia may also be a factor. The arterial pH is usually normal at rest but may increase considerably on exercise as a result of the hyperventilation and consequent respiratory alkalosis (compare Figure 3.3), although metabolic acidosis caused by lactic acid accumulation may also occur in late exercise. In terminal respiratory failure, the pH may fall due to increasing P_{CO_2}.

The diffusing capacity for carbon monoxide is often strikingly reduced in these patients to the neighborhood of 5 mL·min^{-1}·mm Hg^{-1} (normal value 25 to 30 depending on age and stature). This may be a useful diagnostic pointer: if the diffusing capacity is not low, the diagnosis should be regarded with suspicion. The reduction is caused in part by the thickening of the blood–gas barrier (Figure 2.5). In addition, the blood volume of the pulmonary capillaries decreases because many of the vessels are obliterated by the fibrotic process. A further factor in the lower measured diffusing capacity is probably the $\dot{V}_A/\dot{Q}$ inequality, which causes uneven emptying of the lung. The diffusing capacity should not be taken to reflect only the properties of the blood–gas barrier.

Exercise

Patients with mild diffuse interstitial fibrosis may show much more evidence of impaired pulmonary function on exercise than at rest. The changes shown in Figure 3.3B are typical, although this patient had hypersensitivity pneumonitis (see later text). Note that the maximal O_2 intake and CO_2 output were severely limited compared with the normal values of Figure 3.3A. The increase in ventilation on exercise was greatly exaggerated. This exaggeration was chiefly caused by the high rate of breathing, which rose to over 60 breaths per minute during maximal exercise.

As a result of the high ventilation, which was out of proportion to the increase in O_2 uptake and CO_2 output, the alveolar and arterial P_{CO_2} fell and the alveolar P_{O_2} rose. However, as noted earlier, the arterial P_{O_2} fell, thus increasing the alveolar–arterial difference for P_{O_2}. This result can be explained partly by the impaired diffusion characteristics of the lung (Figure 5.8). However, most of the hypoxemia on exercise was caused by $\dot{V}_A/\dot{Q}$ inequality.

One factor that tends to reduce the arterial P_{O_2} on exercise is the abnormal small rise in cardiac output. These patients typically have an increased pulmonary vascular resistance. This is particularly evident on exercise, during which the pulmonary artery pressure may rise substantially. The high resistance is caused by the obliteration of much of the pulmonary capillary bed by the interstitial fibrosis (see Figure 2.5). Another factor is hypertrophy of vascular smooth muscle and consequent narrowing of the small arteries. It is important to appreciate that an abnormally low cardiac output in the presence of $\dot{V}_A/\dot{Q}$ inequality can cause hypoxemia. One way of looking at this is that a low cardiac output results in a low P_{O_2} in the mixed venous blood (see Chapter 9). As a consequence, a lung unit with a given $\dot{V}_A/\dot{Q}$ will oxygenate the blood less than when the mixed venous P_{O_2} is normal.

The importance of this factor can be seen if we consider some results obtained in our laboratory in a patient with interstitial lung disease. During exercise that raised the O_2 uptake from about 300 to 700 mL/min, the arterial P_{O_2} fell from 50 to 35 mm Hg. The rise in cardiac output was only from 4.6 to 5.7 L/min; the normal value for this level of exercise is approximately 10 L/min. As a result, the P_{O_2} in the mixed venous blood fell to 17 mm Hg (normal value is approximately 35 mm Hg). Calculations show that if the cardiac output had increased to 10 L/min (and the pattern of $\dot{V}_A/\dot{Q}$ inequality remained unchanged), the arterial P_{O_2} would have been some 10 mm Hg higher.

If the diffusing capacity for carbon monoxide is measured in these patients during exercise, it typically remains low, whereas it may double or triple in normal subjects.

Control of Ventilation
We have already seen that these patients typically have shallow rapid breathing, especially on exercise. The reason for this is not certain, but it is possible that the pattern is caused by reflexes originating in pulmonary irritant receptors or J (juxtacapillary) receptors. The former lie in the bronchi or in the epithelial lining and may be stimulated by the increased traction on the airways caused by the increased elastic recoil of the lung (Figure 5.6). The J receptors are in the alveolar walls and could be stimulated by the fibrotic changes in the interstitium. No direct evidence of increased activity of either receptor is yet available in humans, but work in experimental animals suggests that these reflexes could cause rapid shallow breathing.

The rapid shallow pattern of breathing reduces the respiratory work in patients with reduced lung compliance. However, it also increases ventilation of the anatomic dead space at the expense of the alveoli, so a compromise must be reached.

Treatment and Outcomes
Diffuse pulmonary fibrosis is an invariably fatal process with the majority of people dying within 5 years of diagnosis. No treatment has been shown to improve mortality although the tyrosine kinase inhibitor, nintedanib, and the

antifibrotic agent, pirfenidone, may slow the rate of decline in lung function and are now increasingly used in these patients. Lung transplantation is often pursued in patients who meet strict eligibility criteria.

Other Types of Parenchymal Restrictive Disease

The changes in pulmonary function in diffuse interstitial pulmonary fibrosis have been dealt with at some length because this disease serves as an example for other forms of parenchymal restrictive disease. These diseases are now considered briefly here, and differences in their pattern of pulmonary function are discussed.

Sarcoidosis

This disease is characterized by the presence of granulomatous tissue having a characteristic histologic appearance. It often occurs in several organs.

Pathology

The characteristic lesion is a noncaseating epithelioid granuloma composed of large histiocytes with giant cells and lymphocytes. This lesion may occur in the lymph nodes, lungs, skin, eyes, liver, spleen, and elsewhere. In advanced pulmonary disease, fibrotic changes in the alveolar walls are seen.

Pathogenesis

This is unknown, although an immunologic basis appears likely. One possibility is that an unknown antigen is recognized by an alveolar macrophage, and this results in the activation of a T lymphocyte and the production of interleukin-2. The activated macrophage may also release various products that stimulate fibroblasts, thus explaining the deposition of fibrous tissue in the interstitium.

Clinical Features

Multiple stages of sarcoidosis can be identified based on the radiographic findings.

- *Stage 0:* There are no findings on plain chest radiography, although a CT scan may show enlarged mediastinal lymph nodes (lymphadenopathy).
- *Stage 1:* There is bilateral hilar adenopathy often with right paratracheal adenopathy (**Figure 5.9**). There are no disturbances of pulmonary function. When accompanied by polyarthralgias and erythema nodosum, this is referred to as Löfgren's syndrome
- *Stage 2:* There is bilateral hilar adenopathy as well as reticular opacities, most significant in the mid and upper zones.
- *Stage 3:* There are reticular opacities in the mid-upper lung zones and shrinking hilar adenopathy.
- *Stage 4:* There is fibrosis, predominantly in the upper lobes. Low lung volumes and traction dilatation are often seen.

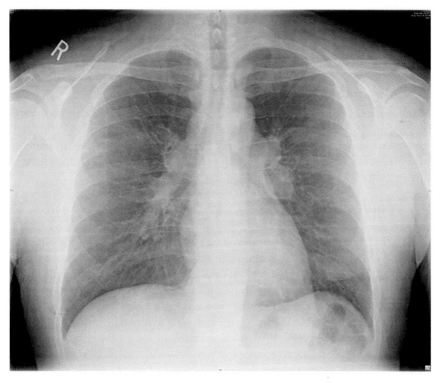

Figure 5.9. Chest radiograph of a patient with stage I sarcoidosis. The radiograph demonstrates bilateral hilar lymphadenopathy but no parenchymal opacities.

Even though multiple stages of the disease are described, patients do not necessarily progress from lower to higher stages. Many patients with lower-stage disease are asymptomatic and are identified as having sarcoidosis when radiographs are performed for other reasons (e.g., employment screening). When present, symptoms typically include dyspnea and a dry unproductive cough. Sarcoidosis can also cause arthritis, uveitis, and parotid gland enlargement as well as a variety of manifestations in the heart and central nervous system.

Pulmonary Function
There is no impairment of function in stages 0 and 1 of the disease. In stages 2 and 3, typical changes of the restrictive type are seen, although the radiographic appearance sometimes suggests more interference with function than actually exists.

Ultimately, significant pulmonary fibrosis may develop, with a severe restrictive pattern of function. All lung volumes are small, but the FEV_1/FVC ratio is preserved. Lung compliance is strikingly reduced, the pressure–volume curve being flattened and shifted downward and to the right (see Figure 3.1).

The resting arterial P_{O_2} is low and often falls considerably on exercise. The arterial P_{CO_2} is normal or low, although, terminally, it may rise as respiratory failure supervenes. The diffusing capacity for carbon monoxide (transfer factor) is reduced significantly. Cor pulmonale may develop in advanced disease.

Treatment

Many patients with lower-stage disease, including those with Löfgren's syndrome, require no treatment and experience spontaneous remission. Treatment, usually with systemic corticosteroids, is initiated in patients with worsening pulmonary function and/or symptoms or extrapulmonary involvement.

Hypersensitivity Pneumonitis

Also referred to as extrinsic allergic alveolitis, hypersensitivity pneumonitis is a parenchymal lung disease that develops as a result of a type 3 (and occasionally type 4) hypersensitivity reaction to inhaled organic dusts. The exposure is usually occupational and heavy but can occur in response to antigens in the home. Precipitins can be demonstrated in the serum.

The term "extrinsic" implies that the etiologic agent is external and can be identified, in contrast to "intrinsic" fibrosing alveolitis (diffuse interstitial fibrosis discussed above), where the cause is unknown. A very large number of exposures have been shown to cause hypersensitivity pneumonitis. Common examples include farmer's lung due to the spores of thermophilic *Actinomyces* in moldy hay, bird breeder's lung caused by avian antigens from feathers and excreta, as well as air-conditioner's lung and bagassosis (in sugarcane workers).

Pathology

The alveolar walls are thickened and infiltrated with lymphocytes, plasma cells, and occasional eosinophils together with collections of histiocytes that, in some areas, form small granulomas. The small bronchioles are usually affected, and there may be exudate in the lumen. Fibrotic changes occur in advanced cases when exposure to the offending antigen persists for long periods of time.

Clinical Features

The disease occurs in either acute or chronic forms. In the former, symptoms of dyspnea, fever, shivering, and cough appear 4 to 6 hours after exposure and continue for 24 to 48 hours. The patient is frequently dyspneic at rest, with fine crepitations throughout both lung fields. The disease may also occur in a chronic form without prior acute attacks. These patients present with progressive dyspnea, usually over a period of years. In the acute form, the chest radiograph may be normal, but frequently micronodular infiltrates are present or ground-glass opacities are seen on CT scans of the chest. In the chronic form, fibrosis of the upper lobes is common and seen on both plain chest radiography and CT scans.

Pulmonary Function

In well-developed disease, the typical restrictive pattern is seen. This includes reduced lung volumes, low compliance, hypoxemia that worsens on exercise, normal or low arterial P_{CO_2}, and a reduced diffusing capacity (Figure 3.3). In the early stages, variable degrees of airway obstruction may be present.

Treatment

The most important treatment principle is elimination of the offending antigen. Some patients require long courses of systemic corticosteroids, but this may not lead to improvement if exposure to the offending antigen continues.

Interstitial Disease Caused by Drugs, Poisons, and Radiation

Various drugs may cause an acute pulmonary reaction, which can proceed to interstitial fibrosis. These drugs include busulfan (used in the treatment of chronic myeloid leukemia), the antibiotic nitrofurantoin, the cardiac antiarrhythmic agent amiodarone, and the cytostatic drug bleomycin. Other antineoplastic drugs can also cause fibrosis. Oxygen in high concentrations following bleomycin administration can cause acute toxic changes with subsequent interstitial fibrosis, even years after the patient received the medication. Ingestion of the weed killer paraquat results in the rapid development of lethal interstitial fibrosis. Therapeutic radiation causes acute pneumonitis followed by fibrosis if lung is included in the field.

Asbestosis

Chronic exposure to asbestos fibers can lead to development of diffuse interstitial fibrosis many years after the exposure. This entity, whose clinical features, pulmonary function, and gas exchange abnormalities resemble idiopathic pulmonary fibrosis, is described further in Chapter 7.

Collagen Vascular Diseases

Interstitial fibrosis with a typical restrictive pattern may be found in patients with systemic sclerosis (generalized scleroderma). Dyspnea is often severe and out of proportion to the changes in radiologic appearance or lung function. Other connective tissue diseases that may produce fibrosis include systemic lupus erythematosus and rheumatoid arthritis.

Lymphangitis Carcinomatosa

This refers to the spread of carcinoma tissue through pulmonary lymphatics and may complicate carcinomas, chiefly of the stomach or breast. Dyspnea is prominent, and the typical restrictive pattern of lung function may be seen.

DISEASES OF THE PLEURA

Pneumothorax

Air can enter the pleural space either from the lung or, less commonly, through the chest wall as a result of a penetrating wound. The pressure in the intrapleural space is normally subatmospheric as a result of the elastic recoil forces of the lung and chest wall. When air enters the space, the lung collapses and the rib cage springs out (see *West's Respiratory Physiology: The Essentials*. 10th ed. p. 121). These changes are evident on a chest radiograph **(Figure 5.10)**, which shows partial or complete collapse of the lung, overexpansion of the rib cage and depression of the diaphragm on the affected side, and sometimes displacement of the mediastinum away from the pneumothorax. These changes are most evident if the pneumothorax is large, particularly if a tension pneumothorax is present (see later text).

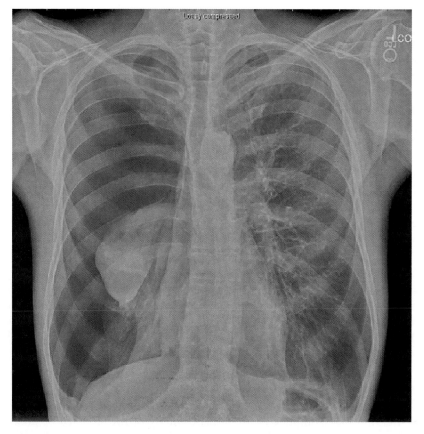

Figure 5.10. Chest radiograph showing a large right-sided spontaneous pneumothorax. Note the small, collapsed right lung.

Spontaneous Pneumothorax

- Can occur in individuals with or without underlying lung diseases.
- Accompanied by sudden onset of dyspnea and pleuritic pain.
- Gradually absorbed by the blood.
- Tube thoracostomy may be required for large pneumothoraces.
- Recurrent attacks may require surgery.
- Tension pneumothorax is a medical emergency.

Spontaneous Pneumothorax

The causes of spontaneous pneumothorax are grouped into two categories. In *primary* spontaneous cases, pneumothorax develops without any predisposing lung disease. Typically occurring in tall young males, this form is caused by the rupture of a small bleb on the surface of the lung near the apex possibly due to the high mechanical stresses that occur in the upper zone of the upright lung (see Figure 3.4). In *secondary* spontaneous cases, the patient has an underlying lung disease such as COPD, cystic fibrosis, or *Pneumocystis* pneumonia that predisposes to pneumothorax. It may also occur during mechanical ventilation with high airway pressures (see Chapter 10).

In either category, the presenting symptom is often sudden, unilateral pleuritic pain accompanied by dyspnea. On auscultation in patients with large pneumothoraces, breath sounds are reduced on the affected side. The diagnosis is readily confirmed by a radiograph and can now be identified using chest ultrasound.

The pneumothorax gradually absorbs because the sum of the partial pressures in the venous blood is considerably less than atmospheric pressure. Tube thoracostomy may be necessary to resolve large pneumothoraces or in patients with underlying lung disease. This involves inserting a tube through the chest wall and connecting the tube to an underwater seal, allowing air to escape from the chest but not to enter it. Recurrent attacks may need surgical treatment to promote adhesions between the two pleural surfaces (pleurodesis).

Tension Pneumothorax

In a small proportion of pneumothoraces, the communication between the lung and the pleural space functions as a check valve. As a consequence, air enters the space during inspiration but cannot escape during expiration. The result is a large pneumothorax in which the pressure may considerably exceed atmospheric pressure and thus interfere with venous return to the thorax.

This medical emergency is recognized by increasing respiratory distress, tachycardia, distended neck veins, and signs of mediastinal shift, such as tracheal deviation and displacement of the apex beat. While chest radiographs demonstrate characteristic changes, diagnosis must often be made on clinical grounds before the radiograph is obtained. Treatment consists of urgently relieving the pressure by inserting a needle through the chest wall on the affected side then performing tube thoracostomy.

Pulmonary Function

As would be expected, a pneumothorax reduces the FEV_1 and FVC, but in practice, pulmonary function tests are rarely performed in the evaluation of acute dyspnea and would not be used in the diagnosis of pneumothorax.

Pleural Effusion

This refers to fluid rather than air in the pleural space. It is not a disease in its own right, but it frequently accompanies serious disease, and an explanation should always be sought.

The patient often reports dyspnea if the effusion is large, and there may be pleuritic pain from the underlying disease. The chest signs are often informative and include reduced movement of the chest on the affected side, absence of breath sounds, and dullness to percussion. Chest radiographs, CT scans, and ultrasound can be used to identify pleural effusions (**Figure 5.11A–C**).

Pleural effusions can be divided into exudates and transudates according to whether their protein content and lactate dehydrogenase concentrations are high or low. Exudates can occur due to a large number of diseases, but the most common causes are malignancies and infections. Transudates complicate severe heart failure and other edematous states such as cirrhosis and chronic kidney disease. While drainage of an effusion leads to symptomatic improvement, treatment should be directed at the underlying cause to

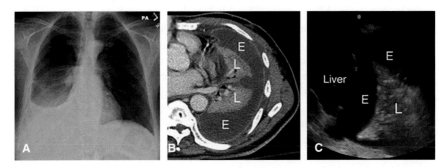

Figure 5.11. Appearance of pleural effusions on chest imaging. Panel A. Plain chest radiograph. Note the dense, homogeneous opacity obscuring the right hemidiaphragm and right heart border. The upper margin of the opacity has a curvilinear appearance, referred to as a "meniscus sign," that is highly suggestive of effusion. **Panel B**. Chest CT scan image. The lung (*L*) is compressed by the surrounding effusion (*E*); **Panel C**. Ultrasound image showing an effusion (*E*), lung (*L*) and liver. The lung is more visible on ultrasound than normal because it is denser due to compression by the surrounding fluid. Note that the fluid is black on ultrasound, unlike on plain chest radiograph.

prevent recurrence. Pulmonary function is impaired as in pneumothorax, but the measurements are not performed in practice.

Variants of pleural effusion include empyema (pyothorax), hemothorax, and chylothorax, which refer to the presence of pus, blood, and lymph, respectively, in the pleural space.

Pleural Thickening

Occasionally, a long-standing pleural effusion results in a rigid, contracted fibrotic pleura that splints the lung and prevents its expansion. This can result in a severe restrictive type of functional impairment, particularly if the disease is bilateral. Surgical stripping may be necessary.

DISEASES OF THE CHEST WALL

Scoliosis

Bony deformity of the chest can cause restrictive disease. "Scoliosis" refers to lateral curvature of the spine and kyphosis to posterior curvature. Scoliosis is more serious, especially if the angulation is high in the vertebral column. It is frequently associated with a backward protuberance of the ribs, giving the appearance of an added kyphosis. In most cases, the cause is unknown, although the condition is occasionally caused by bony tuberculosis or neuromuscular disease.

The patient initially reports dyspnea on exertion; breathing tends to be rapid and shallow. Hypoxemia later develops, and eventually carbon dioxide retention and cor pulmonale may supervene. Bronchitis is common if the patient smokes.

Pulmonary function tests typically show a reduction in all lung volumes. Airway resistance is nearly normal if related to lung volume. However, there is inequality of ventilation, partly because of airway closure in dependent regions. Parts of the lung are compressed and there are often areas of atelectasis.

The hypoxemia is caused by ventilation–perfusion inequality. In advanced disease, a reduced ventilatory response to CO_2 can often be demonstrated. This reduction reflects the increased work of breathing caused by deformity of the chest wall. Not only is the chest wall stiff, but also the respiratory muscles operate inefficiently. The pulmonary vascular bed is restricted, causing a rise in pulmonary artery pressure, which is exaggerated by the alveolar hypoxia. Venous congestion and peripheral edema may develop. The patient may succumb to an intercurrent pulmonary infection or respiratory failure.

Ankylosing Spondylitis

In this disease of unknown etiology, there is a gradual but relentless onset of immobility of the vertebral joints and fixation of the ribs. As a result, the movement of the chest wall is grossly reduced. There is a reduction of FVC and TLC, but the FEV_1/FVC ratio and the airway resistance are normal. The compliance of the chest wall may fall, and there is often some uneven ventilation, probably secondary to the reduced lung volume. While the lung parenchyma remains normal in nearly all cases and diaphragmatic movement is preserved, a small percentage of patients develop fibrosis in the apical regions of the lungs. Respiratory failure does not occur.

NEUROMUSCULAR DISORDERS

Diseases affecting the muscles of respiration or their nerve supply include poliomyelitis, Guillain-Barré syndrome, amyotrophic lateral sclerosis, myasthenia gravis, botulism, and muscular dystrophies (see Table 2.1 and Figure 2.3). All these diseases can lead to dyspnea and respiratory failure. The inability of the patient to take in a deep breath is reflected in a reduced FVC, TLC, inspiratory capacity, and FEV_1. The diffusing capacity for carbon monoxide is typically normal because the lung parenchyma is unaffected.

It should be remembered that the most important muscle of respiration is the diaphragm, and patients with progressive disease often do not report dyspnea until the diaphragm is involved. By then, their ventilatory reserve may be severely compromised. The progress of the disease can be monitored by measuring the FVC and the blood gases. The maximal inspiratory and expiratory pressures that the patient can develop are also reduced. Assisted ventilation (see Chapter 10) may become necessary.

KEY CONCEPTS

1. Diffuse interstitial pulmonary fibrosis is an example of restrictive lung disease characterized by dyspnea, reduced exercise tolerance, small lungs, and reduced lung compliance.

2. The alveolar walls show marked infiltration with collagen and obliteration of capillaries.

3. Airway resistance is not increased; indeed, a forced expiration can result in abnormally high flow rates because of the increased radial traction on the airway.

4. Diffusion of oxygen across the blood–gas barrier is impeded by the thickening and may result in hypoxemia, especially on exercise. However, ventilation–perfusion inequality is the major factor in the impaired gas exchange.

5. Other restrictive disorders are caused by diseases of the pleura or chest wall or neuromuscular disease.

CLINICAL VIGNETTE

A 47-year-old woman is referred to the pulmonary clinic for evaluation of increasing dyspnea on exertion and fatigue. She works as a sales clerk in a department store and is having difficulty at work due to breathlessness with her daily tasks. She has a chronic, nonproductive cough and denies hemoptysis, chest pain, fevers, arthralgias, rash, or ocular symptoms. On physical examination, her S_pO_2 is 93% breathing ambient air. She has end-inspiratory crackles in her bilateral lung fields, normal cardiac abdominal and skin exams, and no clubbing. A chest radiograph is obtained and reveals the following:

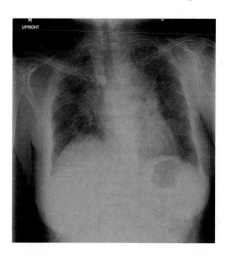

Parameter	Predicted	Prebron-chodilator	% Predicted	Postbron-chodilator	% Change
FVC (L)	2.73	1.53	56	1.59	4
FEV₁ (L)	2.28	1.12	49	1.10	-2
FEV₁/FVC	0.83	0.73	88	0.69	-6

Bronchoscopy is performed and histopathologic examination of samples obtained via transbronchial biopsy reveals noncaseating granulomas.

Questions

- What changes would you expect to see in her TLC and DLCO?
- How will her pressure–volume curve compare to that of a healthy individual?
- If you were to measure her arterial blood gases, what would you expect to find with her acid–base status?
- What will happen to her alveolar–arterial oxygen difference during exercise?

1. A 67-year-old man, who is a lifelong nonsmoker, complains of worsening dyspnea and dry cough over a 6-month period. On exam, he has a fast respiratory rate and is taking small breaths. He has fine crackles (crepitations) in the lower lung zones on auscultation and finger clubbing. A chest radiograph shows low lung volumes and reticulonodular opacities in the bilateral lower lung fields. Which of the following results would you expect to see on pulmonary function testing in this patient?
    A. Increased FEV_1
    B. Increased FVC
    C. Increased FEV_1/FVC ratio
    D. Increased TLC
    E. Increased airway resistance when related to lung volume

2. The arterial hypoxemia of a patient with diffuse interstitial pulmonary fibrosis:
    A. Typically worsens on exercise.
    B. Is chiefly caused by diffusion impairment.
    C. Is associated with a large increase in diffusing capacity during exercise.
    D. Is usually associated with carbon dioxide retention.
    E. Is improved during exercise because of the abnormally large increase in cardiac output.

3. In a patient with diffuse interstitial fibrosis of the lung, the maximal expiratory flow rate at a given lung volume may be higher than in a normal subject because:
    A. Expiratory muscles have a large mechanical advantage.
    B. Airways have a small diameter.
    C. Dynamic compression of the airways is more likely than in a normal subject.
    D. Radial traction on the airways is increased.
    E. Airway resistance is increased.

4. Two patients are referred to the pulmonary diagnostic laboratory on the same day for pulmonary function testing. The first patient has advanced amyotrophic lateral sclerosis (ALS) while the second has idiopathic pulmonary fibrosis. If you were to compare the pulmonary function tests obtained in these two patients, which of the following measurements would you expect to fall within the normal range in the patient with ALS and abnormal range in the patient with pulmonary fibrosis?
    A. Diffusion capacity for carbon monoxide
    B. Forced expiratory volume in 1 second
    C. Forced vital capacity
    D. FEV_1/FVC ratio
    E. Total lung capacity

5. A 59-year-old woman with chronic obstructive pulmonary disease presents to the emergency department after developing the sudden onset of pleuritic left-sided chest pain and dyspnea. While she is being evaluated, she develops worsening dyspnea, tachycardia, and hypotension. On exam, her neck veins are distended, her trachea is deviated to the right, and she has absent breath sounds on the left side of her chest. Which of the following interventions is indicated at this time?

   A. Electrocardiogram
   B. Inhaled bronchodilators
   C. Mechanical ventilatory support
   D. Needle decompression of the left chest
   E. Systemic corticosteroids

6. A 62-year-old woman is evaluated in the pulmonary clinic for a persistent dry cough and worsening dyspnea on exertion over an 18-month period. On exam, her oxygen saturation is 96% breathing air and falls to 90% when she walks around the clinic. She has crepitations on auscultation of the bilateral lower lung fields but no other significant findings. A chest radiograph shows low lung volumes and reticular opacities in the bilateral lower lobes, while a chest CT scan shows honeycombing and alveolar septal thickening in the bilateral lower lobes. Which of the following patterns would you expect to see on pulmonary function testing in this patient?

Choice	FEV_1	FVC	FEV_1/FVC	TLC	DLCO
A	Normal	Normal	Normal	Normal	Normal
B	Normal	Normal	Normal	Normal	Decreased
C	Decreased	Decreased	Decreased	Increased	Decreased
D	Decreased	Decreased	Normal	Decreased	Decreased
E	Decreased	Decreased	Normal	Decreased	Increased

7. A 38-year-old man obtains a chest radiograph as part of a pre-employment screening program. After the radiograph reveals bilateral hilar lymphadenopathy but no parenchymal opacities, he is referred to the pulmonary clinic where he reports no symptoms and has a normal physical examination. He undergoes bronchoscopy with transbronchial biopsies, which reveal noncaseating granulomas. Which of the following is true regarding this patient?

   A. He will likely have an increased arterial P_{CO_2} on arterial blood gas analysis.
   B. He is not at risk for involvement in any other organ systems.
   C. Pulmonary function tests will likely show no impairment.
   D. Spontaneous remission is uncommonly seen with this stage of the disease.
   E. Without treatment, he will develop significant pulmonary fibrosis.

VASCULAR DISEASES

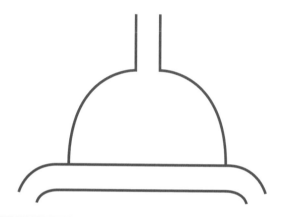

- **Pulmonary Edema**
  Pathophysiology
  Pathogenesis
  Increased Capillary Hydrostatic Pressure
  Increased Capillary Permeability
  Reduced Lymph Drainage
  Decreased Interstitial Pressure
  Decreased Colloid Osmotic Pressure
  Uncertain Etiology
  Clinical Features
  Pulmonary Function
  Mechanics
  Gas Exchange
  Control of Ventilation
  Pulmonary Circulation

- **Pulmonary Embolism**
  Pathogenesis
  Clinical Features
  Medium-Sized Emboli
  Massive Emboli
  Small Emboli

Diagnosis
Pulmonary Function
  Pulmonary Circulation
  Mechanics
  Gas Exchange

- **Pulmonary Hypertension**
  Idiopathic Pulmonary Arterial Hypertension
  Cor Pulmonale

- **Pulmonary Arteriovenous Malformation**

The pathophysiology of the pulmonary vasculature is of great importance. Pulmonary edema is not a disease in its own right, but it complicates many heart and lung diseases and can be life-threatening. Pulmonary embolism is frequently underdiagnosed and may be fatal. The pathophysiology of idiopathic pulmonary arterial hypertension is poorly understood, but recent advances in drug therapy have improved prognosis.

PULMONARY EDEMA

Pulmonary edema is an abnormal accumulation of fluid in the extravascular spaces and tissues of the lung. It is an important complication of a variety of heart and lung diseases and may be life-threatening.

Pathophysiology

Figure 5.1 reminds us that the pulmonary capillary is lined by endothelial cells and surrounded by an interstitial space. As the figure shows, the interstitium is narrow on one side of the capillary, where it is formed by the fusion of the two basement membranes, while on the other side, it is wider and contains type I collagen fibers. This latter region is particularly important for fluid exchange. Between the interstitial and alveolar spaces are the alveolar epithelium, composed predominantly of type 1 cells, and the superficial layer of surfactant (not shown in Figure 5.1).

The capillary endothelium is highly permeable to water and many solutes, including small molecules and ions. Proteins have a restricted movement across the endothelium. By contrast, the alveolar epithelium is much less permeable, and even small ions are largely prevented from crossing by passive diffusion. In addition, the epithelium actively pumps water from the alveolar to interstitial space using a sodium, potassium, ATPase pump.

Hydrostatic forces tend to move fluid out of the capillary into the interstitial space, and osmotic forces tend to keep it in. The movement of fluid across the endothelium is governed by the Starling equation:

$$\dot{Q} = K\left[(P_c - P_i) - \sigma(\pi_c - \pi_i)\right] \qquad \text{(Eq. 6.1)}$$

where $\dot{Q}$ is the net flow out of the capillary; K the filtration coefficient; P_c and P_i the hydrostatic pressures in the capillary and interstitial space, respectively; π_c and π_i the corresponding colloid osmotic pressures; and σ the reflection coefficient. This last variable indicates the effectiveness of the membrane in preventing (reflecting) the passage of proteins compared with that of water across the endothelium, and the coefficient is reduced in diseases that damage the cells and increase the permeability.

Although this equation is valuable conceptually, its practical use is limited. Of the four pressures, only one, the colloid osmotic pressure within the capillary, is known with any certainty. Its value is 25 to 28 mm Hg. The capillary hydrostatic

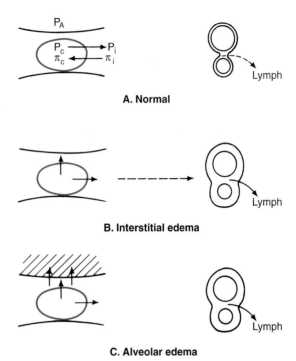

P_A

P_c → P_i
π_c ← π_i

Lymph

A. Normal

Lymph

B. Interstitial edema

Lymph

C. Alveolar edema

Figure 6.1. Stages of pulmonary edema. A. There is normally a small lymph flow from the lung. **B.** Interstitial edema. Here, there is an increased flow with engorgement of the perivascular and peribronchial spaces and some widening of the alveolar wall interstitium. **C.** Some fluid crosses the epithelium, producing alveolar edema.

pressure is probably halfway between arterial and venous pressures but varies markedly from top to bottom of the upright lung. The colloid osmotic pressure of the interstitial fluid is not known but is approximately 20 mm Hg in lung lymph. However, there is some question as to whether this lymph has the same protein concentration as the interstitial fluid around the capillaries. The interstitial hydrostatic pressure is unknown but is thought by some physiologists to be substantially below atmospheric pressure. The value of σ in the pulmonary capillaries is approximately 0.7. It is probable that the net pressure from the Starling equilibrium is outward, causing a lymph flow of perhaps 20 mL/hr.

The fluid that leaves the capillaries moves within the interstitial space of the alveolar wall and tracks to the perivascular and peribronchial interstitium **(Figure 6.1)**. This tissue normally forms a thin sheath around the pulmonary arteries, veins, and bronchi and contains the lymphatics. The alveoli themselves are devoid of lymphatics, but once the fluid reaches the perivascular and peribronchial interstitium, some of it is carried in the lymphatics while some moves through the loose interstitial tissue. The lymphatics actively pump the lymph toward the bronchial and hilar lymph nodes.

If excessive amounts of fluid leak from the capillaries, two factors tend to limit this flow. The first is a fall in the colloid osmotic pressure of the interstitial fluid as the protein is diluted as a result of the faster filtration of water compared with protein. However, this factor does not operate if the permeability of the capillary is greatly increased. The second is a rise in hydrostatic pressure in the interstitial space, which reduces the net filtration pressure. Both factors act to reduce fluid movement out of the capillaries.

Two stages in the formation of pulmonary edema are recognized (Figure 6.1). The first is *interstitial edema*, which is characterized by the engorgement of the perivascular and peribronchial interstitial tissue (cuffing), as shown in **Figure 6.2**. Widened lymphatics can be seen, and lymph flow increases. In addition, some widening of the interstitium of the thick side of the capillary occurs. Pulmonary function is little affected at this stage, and the condition is difficult to recognize, although some radiologic changes may be seen (see later text).

The second stage is *alveolar edema* (**Figure 6.3**). Here, fluid moves across the epithelium into the alveoli, which are filled one by one. As a result of surface tension forces, the edematous alveoli shrink. Ventilation is prevented, and to the extent that the alveoli remain perfused, shunting of blood occurs and hypoxemia is inevitable. The edema fluid may move into the small and large airways and be coughed up as voluminous frothy sputum. The sputum is often pink because of the presence of red blood cells. What prompts the transition from interstitial to alveolar edema is not fully understood, but it may be that the lymphatics become overloaded and that the pressure in

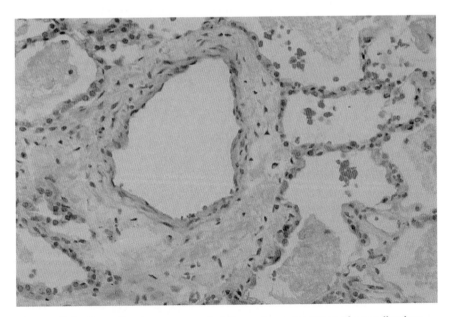

Figure 6.2. **Example of engorgement of the perivascular space of a small pulmonary blood vessel by interstitial edema.** Some alveolar edema is also present. (Image courtesy of Edward Klatt, MD.)

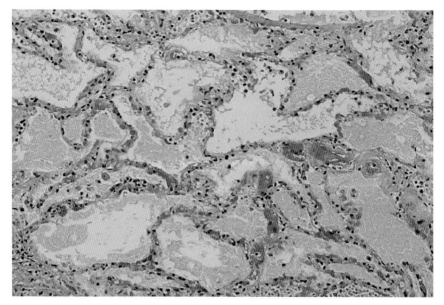

Figure 6.3. Section of human lung showing alveolar edema. (Image courtesy of Edward Klatt, MD.)

the interstitial space increases so much that fluid spills over into the alveoli. Probably, the alveolar epithelium is damaged and its permeability is increased. This would explain the presence of protein and red cells in the alveolar fluid.

Stages of Pulmonary Edema

1. Interstitial edema
   Increased lymph flow from the lung
   Perivascular and peribronchial cuffing
   Septal lines on the chest radiograph
   Little effect on pulmonary function
2. Alveolar edema
   Often severe dyspnea and orthopnea
   Patient may cough up pink, frothy fluid.
   Marked opacification on the radiograph
   Often severe hypoxemia

Pathogenesis

This is best discussed under seven headings, as shown in **Table 6.1**.

Table 6.1	Causes of Pulmonary Edema
Mechanism	**Precipitating Event**
Increased capillary hydrostatic pressure	Myocardial infarction, mitral stenosis, fluid overload, pulmonary venoocclusive disease
Increased capillary permeability	Inhaled or circulating toxins, sepsis, radiation, oxygen toxicity, ARDS
Reduced lymph drainage	Increased central venous pressure, lymphangitic carcinomatosis
Decreased interstitial pressure	Rapid removal of pleural effusion or pneumothorax, hyperinflation
Decreased colloid osmotic pressure	Overtransfusion, hypoalbuminemia
Hypoxic pulmonary vasoconstriction	High altitude
Uncertain etiology	Neurogenic, overinflation, heroin

Increased Capillary Hydrostatic Pressure

This is the most common cause of pulmonary edema and frequently complicates heart disease, such as acute myocardial infarction, hypertensive left ventricular failure, and mitral valve disease. In all these conditions, left atrial pressure rises, causing an increase in pulmonary venous and capillary pressures. This can be recognized at right heart catheterization by measuring the pulmonary arterial wedge pressure (the pressure in a catheter that has been wedged in a small pulmonary artery), which is approximately equal to pulmonary venous pressure.

Whether pulmonary edema occurs in these conditions depends on the rate of rise of the pressure. For example, in patients with mitral stenosis in whom the venous pressure is gradually raised over a period of years, remarkably high values may occur without clinical evidence of edema. This is partly because the caliber or number of the lymphatics increases to accommodate the higher lymph flow. However, these patients often have marked interstitial edema. By contrast, a patient with an acute myocardial infarction or with acute mitral valve failure may develop alveolar edema with a smaller but more sudden rise in pulmonary venous pressure.

Noncardiogenic causes also occur. Edema may be precipitated by excessive intravenous infusions of saline, plasma, or blood, leading to a rise in capillary pressure. Diseases of the pulmonary veins, such as pulmonary venoocclusive diseases, may also result in edema.

The cause of the edema in all these conditions is partly the increase in hydrostatic pressure, which disturbs the Starling equilibrium. However, when the capillary pressure is raised to high levels, ultrastructural changes occur in the capillary walls, including disruption of the capillary endothelium, alveolar epithelium, or sometimes all layers of the wall. The result is an increase in permeability with movement of fluid, protein, and cells into the alveolar spaces. The condition is known as capillary stress failure.

With moderate rises in capillary pressure and consequent disturbance of the Starling equilibrium, the alveolar edema fluid has a low protein concentration because the permeability characteristics of the capillary wall are largely preserved. This is sometimes known as low-permeability edema. Traditionally, this has been contrasted with the alveolar edema that occurs when the capillary permeability has been increased, as discussed in the next section. In this case, large amounts of protein are lost from the capillaries, and therefore, the alveolar fluid has a relatively high protein concentration (high-permeability edema). The edema fluid also typically contains red blood cells, which escape through the damaged capillary walls. However, it is now clear that a sufficiently large increase in capillary pressure can also result in a high-permeability type of edema because of damage to the capillary walls caused by the high pressure, that is, stress failure. In fact, there is a continuous spectrum from low-permeability to high-permeability edema depending on the degree of increase in the pulmonary capillary pressure.

Increased Capillary Permeability

Apart from the situation referred to above, an increased capillary permeability also occurs in a variety of conditions. Toxins that are inhaled (such as chlorine, sulfur dioxide, and nitrogen oxides) or that circulate (such as endotoxin in septic patients) cause pulmonary edema in this way. Therapeutic radiation to the lung may cause edema and, ultimately, interstitial fibrosis. Oxygen toxicity produces a similar picture. Another cause is the acute respiratory distress syndrome (ARDS) (see Chapter 8). As discussed, the edema fluid typically has a high protein concentration and contains many blood cells.

Reduced Lymph Drainage

This can be an exaggerating factor if another cause is present. One of these is an increased central venous pressure, which may occur in ARDS, heart failure, and overtransfusion. This apparently interferes with the normal drainage of the thoracic duct. Another cause is obstruction of lymphatics, as in lymphangitic carcinomatosis.

Decreased Interstitial Pressure

This would be expected to promote edema from the Starling equation, although whether this occurs in practice is uncertain. However, if patients have a large unilateral pleural effusion or pneumothorax and then the lung is rapidly expanded, sometimes pulmonary edema develops on that side, a condition referred to as reexpansion pulmonary edema. This may be partly related to the large mechanical forces acting on the interstitial space as the lung is expanded. However, the edema fluid is of the high-permeability type, and it is probable that the high mechanical stresses in the alveolar walls cause ultrastructural changes in the capillary walls (stress failure).

Decreased Colloid Osmotic Pressure

This is rarely responsible for pulmonary edema on its own, but it can exaggerate the edema that occurs when some other precipitating factor is present. Overtransfusion with saline is an important example. Another example is the hypoproteinemia of the nephrotic syndrome.

Uncertain Etiology

This includes several forms of pulmonary edema. High-altitude pulmonary edema occasionally affects climbers and skiers (**Figure 6.4**). The wedge pressure is normal, so a raised pulmonary venous pressure is not the culprit. However, the pulmonary artery pressure is high because of hypoxic vasoconstriction. Current evidence shows that the arteriolar constriction is uneven and that regions of the capillary bed that are therefore not protected from the high pressure develop the ultrastructural changes of stress failure. This hypothesis would explain the high protein concentration in the alveolar fluid. Treatment is by descent to a lower altitude. When descent is delayed or infeasible, oxygen should be given if it is available while pulmonary vasodilators such as calcium channel blockers and phosphodiesterase inhibitors can be used to lower pulmonary artery pressure.

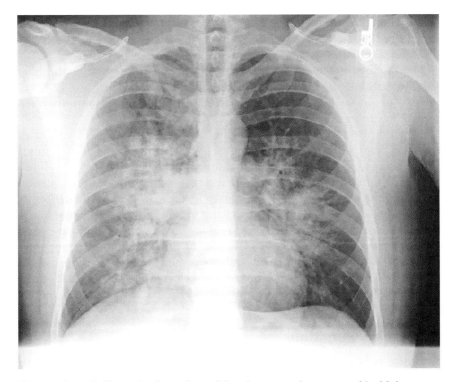

Figure 6.4. Radiograph of a patient with pulmonary edema caused by high altitude. Note the blotchy shadowing, especially on the right side. (Image courtesy of Peter Hackett, MD.)

Neurogenic pulmonary edema is seen after severe central nervous system injuries such as traumatic brain injury or subarachnoid hemorrhage. Again, the mechanism is probably stress failure of pulmonary capillaries because there is a large rise in systemic arterial and pulmonary capillary pressures associated with heightened activity of the sympathetic nervous system.

Overinflation of the lung during mechanical ventilation can cause pulmonary edema likely due to large mechanical forces in the alveolar walls that damage the capillary walls.

Heroin overdose can also complicate overdoses with both injected and orally administered opioids such as heroin and methadone. The mechanism for this is unclear.

Clinical Features

These features depend to some extent on the etiology of the edema, but some generalizations can be made. Dyspnea is usually a prominent symptom; breathing is typically rapid and shallow. Mild edema may cause few symptoms at rest, but exertional dyspnea is inevitable. Orthopnea (increased dyspnea while recumbent) is common, particularly in patients with a cardiac etiology. Paroxysmal nocturnal dyspnea (the patient awakes at night with severe dyspnea and wheezing) and periodic breathing may occur. Cough is frequent and dry in the early stages. However, in fulminant edema, the patient may cough up large quantities of pink foamy sputum. Cyanosis may be present.

On auscultation, fine crepitations are heard on inspiration at the lung bases in early edema. In more severe cases, musical sounds may also be heard because of airway narrowing. Abnormal heart sounds or murmurs are often present in cardiogenic edema.

Depending on the cause of the edema, the chest radiograph may show an enlarged heart and prominent pulmonary vessels. Interstitial edema causes septal lines to appear on the radiograph. Referred to as Kerley B lines, these are short, linear, horizontal markings originating near the pleural surface in the lower zones that are caused by edematous interlobular septa. In more severe edema, blotchy shadowing occurs (Figure 6.4). Sometimes, this shadow radiates from the hilar regions, giving a so-called bat's wing or butterfly appearance. The explanation of this distribution is not clear but may be related to the perivascular and peribronchial cuffing that is particularly noticeable around the large vessels in the hilar region (Figures 6.1 and 6.2).

Pulmonary Function

Extensive pulmonary function tests are seldom carried out on patients with pulmonary edema because they are so sick and the information is not required for treatment. The most important abnormalities are in the areas of mechanics and gas exchange.

Mechanics

Pulmonary edema reduces the distensibility of the lung and moves the pressure–volume curve downward and to the right (compare Figure 3.1). An important factor in this is the alveolar flooding, which causes a reduction in volume of the affected lung units as a result of surface tension forces and reduces their participation in the pressure–volume curve. In addition, interstitial edema per se probably stiffens the lung by interfering with its elastic properties, although it is difficult to obtain clear evidence on this. Edematous lungs require abnormally large expanding pressures during mechanical ventilation and tend to collapse to abnormally small volumes when not actively inflated (see Chapter 10).

Airway resistance is typically increased, especially if some of the larger airways contain edema fluid. Reflex bronchoconstriction due to stimulation of irritant receptors in the bronchial walls may also play a role. It is possible that in the absence of alveolar edema, interstitial edema increases the resistance of small airways as a result of their peribronchial cuff (Figure 6.1). This can be thought of as actually compressing the small airways or, at least, isolating them from the normal traction of the surrounding parenchyma **(Figure 6.5)**. There is some evidence that this mechanism increases the closing volume (Figure 1.10) and thus predisposes to intermittent ventilation of the dependent lung.

Gas Exchange

Interstitial edema has little effect on pulmonary gas exchange. A reduced diffusing capacity has sometimes been attributed to edematous thickening of the blood–gas barrier, but the evidence is meager. It is possible that cuffs of interstitial edema around small airways (Figures 6.1 and 6.5) can cause

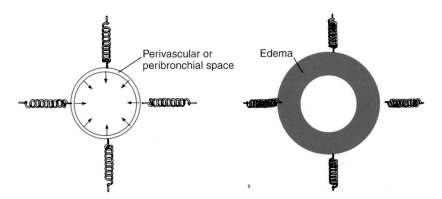

Figure 6.5. Diagram showing how interstitial edema in the perivascular or peribronchial region can reduce the caliber of the vessel or airway. The cuff isolates the structure from the traction of the surrounding parenchyma.

intermittent ventilation of dependent regions of the lung, leading to hypoxemia, but the importance of this in practice is uncertain.

Alveolar edema causes severe hypoxemia chiefly because of blood flow to unventilated units (i.e., shunt; see Figure 10.2). These may be edema-filled alveoli or units supplied by airways that are completely obstructed by fluid. Hypoxic vasoconstriction tends to reduce the true shunt, but often, this is large and may be as much as 50% or more of the pulmonary blood flow in severe edema. Mechanical ventilation with positive end-expiratory pressure (PEEP) often substantially reduces the amount of shunt chiefly by clearing edema fluid from some of the larger airways (see Figure 10.2), although it may not reduce total lung water.

Lung units with low ventilation–perfusion ratios also contribute to the hypoxemia. These presumably lie behind airways that either are partly obstructed by edema fluid or are units in which the ventilation is reduced by their proximity to edematous alveoli. Such lung units are particularly liable to collapse during treatment with oxygen-enriched mixtures (see Figures 9.4 and 9.5), but oxygen therapy is often essential to relieve the hypoxemia. A factor that often aggravates the hypoxemia caused by edema after acute myocardial infarction is a low cardiac output, which reduces the P_{O_2} in mixed venous blood.

The alveolar P_{CO_2} is often normal or low in pulmonary edema because of increased ventilation to the nonedematous alveoli. This is provoked in part by the arterial hypoxemia and also possibly by stimulation of lung receptors (see next section). However, in fulminant pulmonary edema, carbon dioxide retention and respiratory acidosis may develop.

Control of Ventilation

Patients with pulmonary edema typically have rapid, shallow breathing. This may be caused by stimulation of J receptors in the alveolar walls and perhaps other vagal afferents. The rapid breathing pattern minimizes the abnormally high elastic work of breathing. Arterial hypoxemia is an additional stimulus to breathing via the peripheral chemoreceptors.

Pulmonary Circulation

Pulmonary vascular resistance rises, and hypoxic vasoconstriction of poorly ventilated or nonventilated areas is one mechanism for this. In addition, perivascular cuffing probably increases the resistance of the extra-alveolar vessels (Figures 6.2 and 6.5). Other possible factors are the partial collapse of edematous alveoli and alveolar wall edema that may compress or distort capillaries.

The topographical distribution of blood flow is sometimes altered by interstitial edema. The normal apex-to-base gradient becomes inverted, with the result that apical flow exceeds basal (**Figure 6.6**). This is most commonly seen in patients with mitral stenosis. The cause is not fully understood, but it is possible that perivascular cuffs particularly increase the resistance of the lower zone vessels because the lung is less well expanded there (see Figure 3.4).

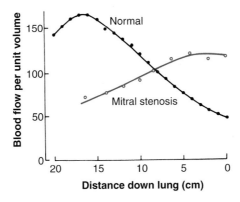

Figure 6.6. Inversion of the topographic distribution of blood flow in a patient with mitral stenosis. The cause is not certain, but interstitial cuffs of edema around the lower zone vessels (Figures 6.2 and 6.5) may be partly responsible.

This inverted distribution is not seen in noncardiogenic forms of edema, such as ARDS.

PULMONARY EMBOLISM

Pulmonary embolism occurs when thrombi form in large veins and travel to the lungs where they become lodged in and occlude the pulmonary circulation. It is associated with significant morbidity and mortality, can be challenging to recognize, and is frequently undiagnosed.

Pathogenesis

The majority of responsible thrombi arise from the deep veins of the lower extremities, but they may also originate in the upper extremities, right side of the heart, and the pelvic veins. Nonthrombotic emboli, such as fat, air, and amniotic fluid, also occur in very specific circumstances but are less common than venous thrombi.

Venous thrombi tend to form in the setting of three important conditions, often referred to as Virchow's triad:

1. Stasis of blood
2. Alterations in the blood coagulation system
3. Abnormalities of the vessel wall (intimal injury)

Stasis of blood is promoted by immobilization following a fracture, severe illness or an operation, local pressure, or venous obstruction. It is common in congestive heart failure, acute spinal cord injury, shock, hypovolemia, dehydration, and varicose veins.

The intravascular *coagulability of blood* is increased in several conditions, such as polycythemia vera and sickle cell disease, which increase the viscosity of the blood leading to sluggish flow next to the vessel wall. A variety of genetic conditions affecting the coagulation cascade are now recognized including factor V Leiden deficiency, antithrombin 3 deficiency, and protein C deficiency. Other conditions, including widespread malignancy, pregnancy, and the use of oral contraceptives, are also associated with hypercoagulability, but the mechanism for these changes is not entirely clear. Aside from genetic and other testing to identify some of the hypercoagulable states listed above, there is no reliable test of an increased tendency for intravascular coagulation.

The *vessel wall may be damaged* by local trauma or by inflammation. This is a common mechanism for venous thrombi following pelvic and lower extremity fractures, for example. Where there is marked local phlebitis with tenderness, redness, warmth, and swelling, the clot may be more securely adherent to the wall.

The presence of thrombosis in the deep veins of the legs or pelvis is often unsuspected until embolism occurs. Sometimes, there is swelling of the limb or local tenderness, and there may be signs of inflammation. Acute dorsiflexion of the ankle may elicit calf pain. Duplex ultrasonography of the upper and lower extremities is used to confirm the presence of deep venous thrombosis but is not effective for examining the iliac or pelvic veins.

When the thrombus fragment is released, it is rapidly swept into one of the pulmonary arteries. While very large thrombi become lodged in a large artery, the thrombus may break up and block several smaller vessels. The lower lobes are frequently involved because they have a high blood flow (see Figure 3.4).

Pulmonary infarction, that is, death of the embolized tissue, occurs infrequently. More often, there is distal hemorrhage and atelectasis, but the alveolar structures remain viable. Depletion of alveolar surfactant may contribute to these changes. Infarction is more likely if the embolus completely blocks a large artery or if there is pre-existing lung or heart disease. Infarction results in alveolar filling with extravasated red cells and inflammatory cells and causes an opacity on the radiograph. Rarely, the infarct becomes infected, leading to an abscess. The infrequency of infarction can be explained, in part, by the fact that most emboli do not obstruct the vessel completely. In addition, bronchial artery anastomoses, and the airways supply oxygen to the lung parenchyma.

Clinical Features

The presentation depends considerably on the size of the embolus and the patient's pre-existing cardiopulmonary status.

Medium-Sized Emboli

These often present with acute onset of pleuritic pain accompanied by dyspnea and, less commonly, slight fever, and cough productive of blood-streaked sputum. Tachycardia is common, and on auscultation, there may be a pleural friction rub. A small pleural effusion may develop. Embolism may mimic pneumonia, although the two entities can typically be distinguished by the rapidity of symptom onset, which is faster for pulmonary embolism.

Massive Emboli

These may produce sudden hemodynamic collapse with shock, pallor, central chest pain, and sometimes loss of consciousness or cardiac arrest. The pulse is rapid and weak, the blood pressure is low, and the neck veins are engorged. The electrocardiogram may show the pattern of right ventricular strain.

Small Emboli

These are frequently unrecognized or only detected as an incidental finding on chest imaging studies performed to evaluate other problems. Repeated small emboli can gradually obliterate the pulmonary capillary bed, resulting in pulmonary hypertension (described further below).

Features of Pulmonary Embolism for Different-Sized Emboli

Small emboli
Frequently unrecognized
Repeated emboli may result in pulmonary hypertension.

Medium-sized emboli
Sometimes pleuritic pain, dyspnea, and slight fever
Cough may produce blood-stained sputum.
May produce pleural friction rub
Chest radiograph is often normal or nearly so.
Lung scan shows unperfused regions.

Massive emboli
Hemodynamic collapse with shock, pallor, and central chest pain
Hypotension with rapid, weak pulse and neck vein engorgement
Sometimes fatal

Diagnosis

Due to the wide variability in clinical presentation, pulmonary embolism can be very difficult to diagnose. Chest radiography is typically unrevealing, although in rare cases, peripheral wedge-shaped opacities suggestive of infarction or areas of decreased vascular markings (oligemia) may be seen. Contrast-enhanced CT scans of the chest are the most commonly used diagnostic test,

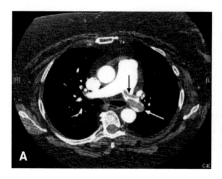 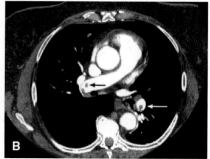

Figure 6.7. Examples of pulmonary emboli on contrast-enhanced CT scan of the chest. Emboli are detected by showing areas where contrast does not fill the pulmonary vasculature, referred to as a "filling defect." **A.** The *black arrow* points to a filling defect in the proximal left main pulmonary artery while the *white arrow* points to a filling defect further out in the left main pulmonary artery. **B.** The *black arrow* points to a filling defect in the right main pulmonary artery while the *white arrow* demonstrates a filling defect in the left lower lobe pulmonary artery.

with the key finding being the presence of filling defects in the pulmonary vasculature **(Figure 6.7)**. For patients who cannot undergo CT scanning due to the risk of contrast administration, lung scans can be made after injecting radiolabeled albumin aggregates into the venous circulation and comparing the distribution of perfusion with the distribution of ventilation measured following inhalation of a radiolabeled aerosol **(Figure 6.8)**. Pulmonary angiography is considered the diagnostic gold standard but is not widely used due to the invasiveness of the procedure and the increasing quality of CT scans.

Pulmonary Function

Pulmonary Circulation

This normally has a large reserve capacity because many capillaries are unfilled. When the pulmonary artery pressure rises, for example, on exercise, these capillaries are recruited and, in addition, some capillary distention occurs. This reserve means that at least half of the pulmonary circulation can be obstructed by an embolus before there is a substantial rise in pulmonary artery pressure.

In addition to the purely mechanical effects of the embolus, there is some evidence that active vasoconstriction occurs, at least for some minutes after embolization **(Figure 6.9)**. The mechanism is not understood, but in experimental animals, local release of serotonin from platelets associated with the embolus has been implicated, as well as reflex vasoconstriction via the sympathetic nervous system. It is not known to what extent these factors operate in humans.

If the embolus is large and if the pulmonary artery pressure rises considerably, the right ventricle may begin to fail. The end-diastolic pressure increases,

VENTILATION
R   L

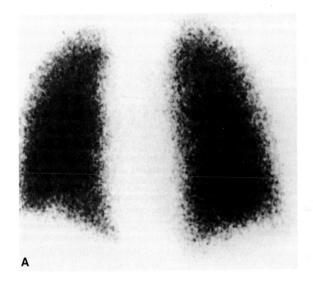

A

PERFUSION
R   L

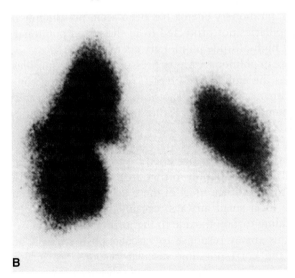

B

Figure 6.8. Lung scan in a patient with multiple pulmonary emboli. A. The ventilation image (made with xenon-133) shows a normal pattern. **B.** The perfusion image (made with technetium-99m albumin) shows areas of absent blood flow in both lungs.

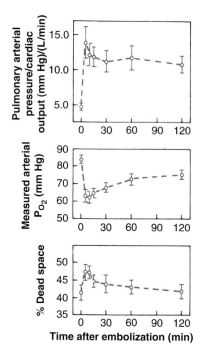

Figure 6.9. Transient changes in pulmonary artery pressure (related to cardiac output), arterial P_{CO_2}, and physiologic dead space in dogs following experimental thromboembolism. These suggest active responses of the pulmonary circulation and airways. The importance of these mechanisms in humans is unknown. (From Dantzker DR, Wagner PD, Tornabene VW, Alzaraki NP, West JB. Gas exchange after pulmonary thromboembolization in dogs. *Circ Res* 1978;42:92–103.)

arrhythmias may develop, and the tricuspid valve may become incompetent. In a few cases, pulmonary edema has been seen, presumably due to leakage from those capillaries not protected from the raised pulmonary artery pressure (compare high-altitude pulmonary edema).

The increase in pulmonary artery pressure gradually subsides over the subsequent days as the embolus resolves. This occurs both through fibrinolysis and through organization of the clot into a small fibrous scar attached to the vessel wall. Patency of the vessel is thus usually restored.

Mechanics

When a pulmonary artery is occluded by a catheter in humans and experimental animals, the ventilation to that area of lung is reduced. The mechanism appears to be a direct effect of the reduced alveolar P_{CO_2} on the smooth muscle of the local small airways, causing bronchoconstriction. It can be reversed by adding carbon dioxide to the inspired gas.

Although this airway response to vascular obstruction is generally much weaker than the corresponding vascular response to airway obstruction (hypoxic vasoconstriction), it serves a similar homeostatic role. The reduction in airflow to the unperfused lung reduces the amount of wasted ventilation and thus the physiologic dead space. This mechanism is apparently short-lived or ineffective after pulmonary thromboembolism in humans because most measurements of the distribution of ventilation with radioactive xenon made some hours after the episode show no defect in the embolized area. However, in experimental animals, transient changes in alveolar P_{O_2}, physiologic dead space, and airway resistance often occur after thromboembolism (Figure 6.9).

The elastic properties of the embolized region may change some hours after the event. In experimental animals, ligation of one pulmonary artery is followed by patchy hemorrhagic edema and atelectasis in the affected lung within 24 hours. This has been attributed to the loss of pulmonary surfactant, which has a rapid turnover and apparently cannot be replenished in a lung that has lost its pulmonary blood flow. Again, it is not yet clear how often this occurs in human pulmonary thromboembolism or whether it is part of the pathological process that has been traditionally called infarction. The fact that most emboli do not completely block the vessel presumably limits its occurrence.

Gas Exchange

Moderate hypoxemia without carbon dioxide retention is often seen after pulmonary embolism. Both the physiologic shunt and dead space are increased. Various explanations for the hypoxemia have been advanced, including diffusion impairment in areas with ongoing blood flow and therefore reduced transit time (see Figure 2.4), opening up of latent pulmonary artery–vein anastomoses as a consequence of the high pulmonary artery pressure and blood flow through infarcted areas.

Measurements by the multiple inert gas elimination technique show that the hypoxemia can be explained by ventilation–perfusion inequality. **Figure 6.10** shows distributions from two patients after massive pulmonary embolism. The most striking features are the large shunts (blood flow to unventilated alveoli) of 20% and 39% and the existence of lung units with high ventilation–perfusion ratios. The latter feature can be explained by the embolized regions where the blood flow is typically greatly reduced but not abolished completely. The precise mechanism of the shunts is not certain, but it may be blood flow through the areas of hemorrhagic atelectasis.

Hypoxemia can also develop due to redistribution of blood flow to the non-embolized areas of the lung. Because the entire cardiac output must traverse the pulmonary circulation, blood that would normally go through occluded regions must now travel through other lung units thus reducing their ventilation–perfusion ratio and depressing the arterial P_{O_2}.

The arterial P_{CO_2} after pulmonary embolism is maintained at the normal level by increasing the ventilation to the alveoli (see Figure 2.9). The increase in ventilation may be substantial because of the large physiologic dead space, and therefore wasted ventilation, caused by the embolized areas.

Some investigators have suggested that the difference in P_{CO_2} between arterial blood and end-tidal gas may indicate pulmonary embolism. The mixed alveolar P_{CO_2} tends to be low because of the high $\dot{V}_A/\dot{Q}$ in the embolized region, and because there is little uneven ventilation in this disease, the end-tidal P_{CO_2} is a useful measure of the mixed alveolar value. However, this test is not generally used.

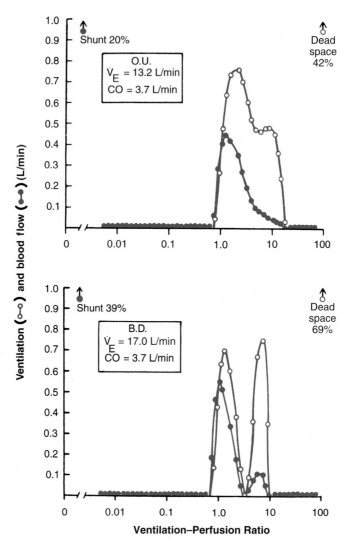

Figure 6.10. Distributions of ventilation–perfusion ratios in two patients with acute massive pulmonary embolism. Note that in both instances, the hypoxemia could be explained by large shunts (blood flow to unventilated lung). In addition, there was a large increase in ventilation to lung units with abnormally high ventilation–perfusion ratios representing the embolized regions. (From D'Alonzo GE, Bower JS, DeHart P, Dantzker DR. The mechanisms of abnormal gas exchange in acute massive pulmonary embolism. *Am Rev Respir Dis* 1983;128:170–172.)

PULMONARY HYPERTENSION

The normal mean pulmonary artery pressure is approximately 15 mm Hg; an increased level (>25 mm Hg) is called pulmonary hypertension.

Three principal mechanisms are as follows:

1. *Increase in Pulmonary Vascular Resistance.* This is the most common cause of severe pulmonary hypertension and can develop due to one of several mechanisms.

   a. A variety of diseases cause structural changes in the blood vessels including medial hypertrophy, intimal thickening, and plexiform lesions. These occur in the pulmonary arterioles and lead to narrowing of the vessels and increased resistance. This is the primary mechanism in patients with idiopathic pulmonary arterial hypertension (see below) as well as pulmonary hypertension seen in patients with scleroderma, systemic lupus erythematosus, cirrhosis, human immunodeficiency virus, and methamphetamine abuse.

   b. Vasoconstriction, principally because of alveolar hypoxia as occurs at high altitude. This is also a component in pulmonary hypertension seen in severe obstructive lung disease or the obesity hypoventilation syndrome.

   c. Vascular obstruction, as in thromboembolism. In addition, the vessels may be occluded by circulating fat, air, amniotic fluid, or cancer cells. Some cases may be caused by repeated small emboli. In schistosomiasis, the parasites lodge in small arteries and cause a granulomatous reaction. A similar phenomenon can occur when talc particles contaminate illicit substances injected by drug users.

   d. Obliteration of the pulmonary capillary bed, as in emphysema or idiopathic pulmonary fibrosis (see Figures 4.2 and 4.3). Various forms of arteritis can also occur, such as in polyarteritis nodosa. Rarely, the small veins are involved, as in pulmonary venoocclusive disease.

2. *Increase in Left Atrial Pressure.* Examples are mitral stenosis and left ventricular failure. Although the changes in pulmonary artery pressure are due to a high pressure in the left atrium, sustained increases in pressure can cause structural changes in the walls of the small pulmonary arteries, including medial hypertrophy and intimal thickening.

3. *Increase in Pulmonary Blood Flow.* This occurs in congenital heart disease with left-to-right shunts through ventricular or atrial septal defects or a patent ductus arteriosus. Initially, the rise in pulmonary artery pressure is relatively small because of the ability of the pulmonary capillaries to accommodate high flows by recruitment and distention. However, sustained high flows result in structural changes in the walls of the small arteries, and eventually, the pulmonary artery pressures may reach systemic levels, causing some right-to-left shunting and arterial hypoxemia (Eisenmenger syndrome).

If the clinical picture suggests pulmonary hypertension, echocardiography is typically performed to estimate the pulmonary artery systolic pressure by determining the amount of regurgitation through the tricuspid valve. Right heart catheterization is the gold standard for measuring pulmonary artery pressure but is invasive and often not required. Once pulmonary hypertension is confirmed on these tests, additional testing is done to determine the etiology, which serves as a guide for treatment.

Idiopathic Pulmonary Arterial Hypertension

This is an uncommon disorder of uncertain cause, although in some cases a genetic predisposition is present. Pulmonary artery pressure is increased due to increased pulmonary vascular resistance resulting from medial hypertrophy, intimal thickening, and plexiform arteriopathy **(Figure 6.11)**. It typically occurs in young to middle-aged women and usually presents with dyspnea on exertion, although in more severe cases, syncope or chest pain on exertion may occur. Examination reveals signs of right ventricular hypertrophy that are confirmed by the ECG and chest radiography. Patients often have hypoxemia, particularly on exertion, and a decrease in the diffusing capacity for carbon monoxide. Left untreated, the disease progresses inexorably and is associated with very high mortality within just a few years. Recent advances in pharmacologic therapy, however, including the use of oral and

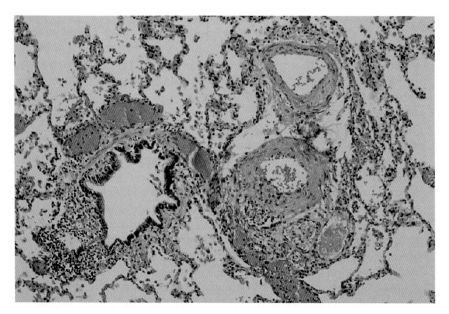

Figure 6.11. Section of human lung obtained on autopsy from a patient with idiopathic pulmonary arterial hypertension. Note the increased thickness of the wall of the arterioles due to smooth muscle hypertrophy. The vessel lumen is narrowed leading to increased vascular resistance. (Image courtesy of Edward Klatt, MD.)

intravenous pulmonary vasodilators, have led to significant improvements in patient outcomes.

Cor Pulmonale

This term refers to right heart disease secondary to primary disease of the lung. The occurrence of right ventricular hypertrophy and fluid retention in COPD was discussed in Chapter 4. The same findings may occur late in restrictive lung disease.

The various factors that lead to pulmonary hypertension include obliteration of the capillary bed by the destruction of alveolar walls or interstitial fibrosis; obstruction by thromboemboli, hypoxic vasoconstriction, and hypertrophy of smooth muscle in the walls of the small arteries; and increased viscosity of the blood caused by polycythemia. Whether the term "right heart failure" should be applied to all these patients is disputed. In some, the output of the heart is increased because it is operating high on the Starling curve, and the output can increase further on exercise. The principal physiological abnormality in these patients is fluid retention. However, in others, true failure develops. Some physicians restrict the term cor pulmonale to those patients who have ECG evidence of right ventricular hypertrophy.

PULMONARY ARTERIOVENOUS MALFORMATION

This uncommon condition is characterized by an abnormal communication between a branch of a pulmonary artery and vein. Most patients have hereditary hemorrhagic telangiectasia. As implied by the name of the disease, these patients also have telangiectasias of the skin or mucous membranes, suggesting the presence of a general vascular defect, and often have a personal or family history of recurrent epistaxis or gastrointestinal bleeding due to vascular abnormalities on those mucosal surfaces as well. In addition to telangiectasias, some patients have finger clubbing and a bruit may be detected on auscultation over the fistula.

Small lesions cause no functional disturbances, whereas larger fistulae cause true shunts and hypoxemia. The arterial P_{O_2} is depressed far below the expected value during oxygen breathing (see Figure 2.6). Untreated arteriovenous malformations also increase the risk of cerebrovascular accidents and intracerebral abscess due to the loss of the filter function of the pulmonary capillary network. While large arteriovenous malformations can be seen on plain chest radiography, contrast-enhanced CT scans are the preferred diagnostic test.

KEY CONCEPTS

1. Fluid movement across the pulmonary capillary endothelium is determined by the Starling equation and disturbances of the normal equilibrium can result in pulmonary edema. A common cause is an increase in capillary pressure as a result of left heart failure.

2. Clinical features of pulmonary edema include dyspnea, orthopnea, cough with blood-stained sputum, tachycardia, and rales on auscultation.

3. Two stages of pulmonary edema are recognized: interstitial and alveolar. The first is difficult to detect, but the second causes major symptoms and signs.

4. Pulmonary embolism is frequently undiagnosed. Medium-sized emboli typically cause pleuritic pain, dyspnea, and cough with blood-streaked sputum. Diagnosis can be made using a CT pulmonary angiogram or a ventilation–perfusion scan. Multiple small emboli can result in pulmonary hypertension.

5. Pulmonary hypertension can be caused by an elevated venous pressure as in left heart failure, an increase in pulmonary blood flow as in some congenital heart diseases, or an increase in pulmonary vascular resistance as, at high altitude, following thromboembolism or loss of capillaries as in emphysema. Another cause is idiopathic pulmonary arterial hypertension.

CLINICAL VIGNETTE

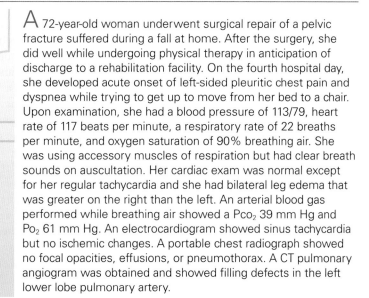

A 72-year-old woman underwent surgical repair of a pelvic fracture suffered during a fall at home. After the surgery, she did well while undergoing physical therapy in anticipation of discharge to a rehabilitation facility. On the fourth hospital day, she developed acute onset of left-sided pleuritic chest pain and dyspnea while trying to get up to move from her bed to a chair. Upon examination, she had a blood pressure of 113/79, heart rate of 117 beats per minute, a respiratory rate of 22 breaths per minute, and oxygen saturation of 90% breathing air. She was using accessory muscles of respiration but had clear breath sounds on auscultation. Her cardiac exam was normal except for her regular tachycardia and she had bilateral leg edema that was greater on the right than the left. An arterial blood gas performed while breathing air showed a Pco_2 39 mm Hg and Po_2 61 mm Hg. An electrocardiogram showed sinus tachycardia but no ischemic changes. A portable chest radiograph showed no focal opacities, effusions, or pneumothorax. A CT pulmonary angiogram was obtained and showed filling defects in the left lower lobe pulmonary artery.

Questions

- What risk factor(s) predisposed the patient to this problem?
- If you were to perform echocardiography, what changes would you expect to see with her pulmonary artery pressure and right heart function?
- How do you account for the fact that she has a normal Pa_{CO_2} on her arterial blood gas?
- What is the mechanism for the patient's hypoxemia?

QUESTIONS

1. Increased movement of fluid from the lumen of pulmonary capillaries into the interstitium can be caused by:
   A. Increased permeability of the alveolar epithelial cells.
   B. Reduced capillary hydrostatic pressure.
   C. Reduced colloid osmotic pressure of the blood.
   D. Increased hydrostatic pressure in the interstitial space.
   E. Reduced colloid osmotic pressure of the interstitial fluid.

2. Concerning the blood–gas barrier in the normal lung:
   A. Fluid can drain through the interstitium of the thick side of the blood–gas barrier.
   B. The alveolar epithelium has a high permeability for water.
   C. The strength of the barrier on the thin side is mainly attributable to the endothelial cells.
   D. No protein normally crosses the capillary endothelium.
   E. Water is actively transported into the alveolar spaces by alveolar epithelial cells.

3. Which of the following statements is true regarding the earliest stages of pulmonary edema?
   A. Fluid tracks through the interstitium of the thin side of the blood–gas barrier to the perivascular and peribronchial spaces.
   B. There is no increase in lung lymph flow.
   C. Fluid floods the alveoli one by one.
   D. The hydrostatic pressure in the interstitium probably falls.
   E. Cuffs of fluid collect around the small arteries and veins.

4. Interstitial pulmonary edema (in the absence of alveolar edema) typically results in:
   A. Septal lines on the chest radiograph.
   B. Increased lung compliance.
   C. Reduced lymph flow from the lungs.
   D. Severe hypoxemia.
   E. Fluffy shadowing on the chest radiograph.

5. Concerning severe pulmonary edema with alveolar filling:
   A. Lung compliance is increased.
   B. Airway resistance is not affected.
   C. The arterial hypoxemia cannot be abolished by breathing 100% oxygen.
   D. Respiration is deep and labored.
   E. The alveolar edema causes chest pain.

6. Moderately large pulmonary emboli often cause:
   A. CO_2 retention.
   B. Increased physiologic dead space.
   C. Pulmonary hypotension.
   D. Rhonchi.
   E. Increased cardiac output.

7. A 41-year-old man presents with a sudden onset of severe dyspnea accompanied by pleuritic left-sided chest pain that began several hours after a transoceanic flight. There is no fever, cough, or hemoptysis. On examination, he has clear breath sounds on auscultation and a normal cardiac examination but leg edema that is greater on the right than the left. Which is the most appropriate initial diagnostic test?
   A. Bronchoscopy
   B. CT of the chest with contrast
   C. Echocardiogram
   D. Pulmonary angiography
   E. Spirometry

8. A 61-year-old woman with no history of smoking is admitted to the hospital with 2 days of worsening dyspnea and a nonproductive cough. On examination, her blood pressure was normal, and she had an elevated jugular venous pulsation, a third heart sound, no murmurs, diffuse crepitations on lung auscultation, and bilateral leg edema. A chest radiograph showed cardiomegaly and diffuse bilateral opacities, while an echocardiogram performed shortly following admission showed a dilated left ventricle with a low ejection fraction of 30% and an increased estimated pulmonary artery systolic pressure of 50 mm Hg. Which of the following most likely accounts for her pulmonary hypertension?
   A. Granulomatous inflammation in the pulmonary arterioles
   B. Left heart failure
   C. Increased pulmonary blood flow
   D. Medial hypertrophy and intimal thickening of the pulmonary arterioles
   E. Occlusion of the pulmonary vascular bed by recurrent thromboemboli

9. A previously healthy 22-year-old man in a high-altitude mountain hut at 4,500 m for 3 days develops severe dyspnea with minimal exertion and a cough productive of pink-tinged sputum. His oxygen saturation by pulse oximetry is found to be abnormally low. Auscultation reveals bilateral crackles in both lungs. Which of the following mechanisms is most likely responsible for this man's condition?
   A. Decreased colloid osmotic pressure
   B. Decreased interstitial pressure
   C. Increased left atrial pressure
   D. Endotoxin-mediated increase in capillary permeability
   E. Exaggerated hypoxic pulmonary vasoconstriction

10. A 57-year-old man with known very severe COPD who continues to smoke cigarettes presents to his doctor with increasing weight gain and bilateral lower leg edema over several weeks. On examination, he has an elevated jugular venous pulsation and bilateral lower leg edema that extend to his knees. An electrocardiogram shows right ventricular hypertrophy and right axis deviation. Which of the following is the most appropriate diagnostic test at this time?
    A. Bronchoscopy
    B. CT scan of the chest without contrast
    C. Echocardiography
    D. Spirometry
    E. Duplex ultrasonography of the lower extremities

ENVIRONMENTAL, NEOPLASTIC, AND INFECTIOUS DISEASES

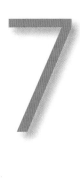

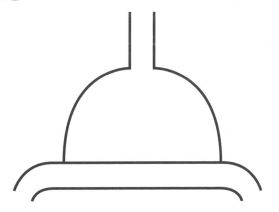

- **Diseases Caused by Inhaled Particles**
  Atmospheric Pollutants
    Carbon Monoxide
    Nitrogen Oxides
    Sulfur Oxides
    Hydrocarbons
    Particulate Matter
    Photochemical Oxidants
    Cigarette Smoke
  Deposition of Aerosols in the Lung
    Impaction
    Sedimentation
    Diffusion
  Clearance of Deposited Particles
    Mucociliary System
    Alveolar Macrophages
  Coal Workers' Pneumoconiosis
    Pathology
    Clinical Features
    Pulmonary Function
  Silicosis
    Pathology
    Clinical Features
    Pulmonary Function
  Asbestos-Related Diseases

Other Pneumoconioses
Byssinosis
Occupational Asthma
- **Neoplastic Diseases**
  Bronchial Carcinoma
    Pathogenesis
    Classification
    Clinical Features
    Pulmonary Function
- **Infectious Diseases**
  Pneumonia
    Pathology
    Clinical Features
    Pulmonary Function
  Tuberculosis
  Fungus Infections
  Pulmonary Involvement in HIV
- **Suppurative Diseases**
  Bronchiectasis
    Pathology
    Clinical Features
    Pulmonary Function
  Cystic Fibrosis
    Pathology
    Clinical Features
    Pulmonary Function

DISEASES CAUSED BY INHALED PARTICLES

Many occupational and industrial lung diseases are caused by inhaled dusts. Atmospheric pollutants are also important factors in the etiology of other diseases, such as chronic bronchitis, emphysema, asthma, and bronchial carcinoma, so we will start by looking at the environment in which we all live.

Atmospheric Pollutants

Carbon Monoxide

This is the largest pollutant by weight in the United States (**Figure 7.1**, *left*). It is produced by the incomplete combustion of carbon in fuels, chiefly in the automobile engine (Figure 7.1, *right*). The main hazard of carbon monoxide is its propensity to tie up hemoglobin. Because carbon monoxide has more than 200 times the affinity of oxygen, it competes successfully with this gas for hemoglobin-binding sites. Carbon monoxide also increases the oxygen affinity of the remaining hemoglobin with the result that it does not release its oxygen so readily to the tissues (see *West's Respiratory Physiology: The Essentials*. 10th ed. p. 92). A commuter using a busy urban freeway may have 5–10% of his hemoglobin bound to carbon monoxide, particularly if he is a cigarette smoker. There is evidence that this can impair cognitive skills. The emission of carbon monoxide and other pollutants by automobile engines can be reduced by installing a catalytic converter that processes the exhaust gases.

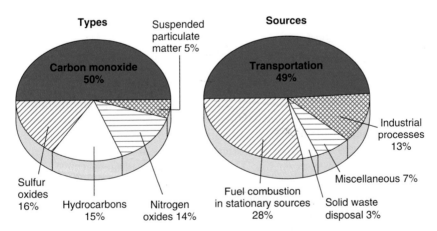

Figure 7.1. **Air pollutants (by weight) in the United States.** Transportation sources, especially automobiles, account for the largest amount of pollutants. Stationary sources, particularly power stations, account for 28%. (From the Environmental Protection Agency.)

Nitrogen Oxides

These are produced when fossil fuels (coal, oil) are burned at high temperatures in power stations and automobiles. These gases cause inflammation of the eyes and upper respiratory tract during smoggy conditions. At higher concentrations, they can cause acute tracheitis, acute bronchitis, and pulmonary edema. The yellow haze of smog is a result of these gases.

Sulfur Oxides

These are corrosive, poisonous gases produced when sulfur-containing fuels are burned, chiefly by power stations. These gases cause inflammation of the mucous membranes, eyes, upper respiratory tract, and bronchial mucosa. Short-term exposure to high concentrations causes pulmonary edema. Long-term exposure to lower levels results in chronic bronchitis in experimental animals. The best way to reduce emissions of sulfur oxides is to use low-sulfur fuels, but these are expensive.

Hydrocarbons

Hydrocarbons, like carbon monoxide, represent unburned wasted fuel. They are not toxic at concentrations normally found in the atmosphere. However, they are hazardous because they form photochemical oxidants under the influence of sunlight (discussed later).

Particulate Matter

This includes particles with a wide range of sizes, up to visible smoke and soot. Major sources are power stations and industrial plants. Often, emission of polluting particles can be reduced by processing the waste air stream by filtering or scrubbing, although removing the smallest particles is often expensive.

Photochemical Oxidants

These include ozone and other substances, such as peroxyacetyl nitrates, aldehydes, and acrolein. They are not primary emissions but are produced by the action of sunlight on hydrocarbons and nitrogen oxides. These reactions are slow with the result that the concentration of the photochemical oxidants may increase several kilometers from where the oil was released. Photochemical oxidants cause inflammation of the eyes and respiratory tract, damage to vegetation, and offensive odors. In higher concentrations, ozone causes pulmonary edema. These oxidants contribute to the thick haze of smog.

The concentration of atmospheric pollutants is often greatly increased by a temperature inversion, that is, a low layer of cold air beneath warmer air. This prevents the normal escape of warm surface air with its pollutants to the upper atmosphere. The deleterious effects of a temperature inversion are particularly marked in a low-lying area surrounded by hills, such as the Los Angeles basin.

Major Atmospheric Pollutants

- Carbon monoxide
- Nitrogen oxides
- Sulfur oxides
- Hydrocarbons
- Particulate matter
- Photochemical oxidants

Cigarette Smoke

This is one of the most important pollutants in practice because it is inhaled by devotees in concentrations many times greater than the pollutants in the atmosphere. It includes approximately 4% carbon monoxide, enough to raise the carboxyhemoglobin level in a smoker's blood to 10%, a percentage sufficient to impair exercise and cognitive performance. The smoke also contains the alkaloid nicotine, which stimulates the autonomic nervous system, causing tachycardia, hypertension, and sweating. Aromatic hydrocarbons and other substances, loosely called "tars," are apparently responsible for the high risk of bronchial carcinoma in cigarette smokers. A male who smokes 35 cigarettes per day has 40 times the risk of a nonsmoker. Increased risks of chronic bronchitis, emphysema, coronary artery disease, and peripheral arterial disease are also well documented. A single cigarette causes a marked increase in airway resistance in many smokers and nonsmokers (see Figure 3.2).

Deposition of Aerosols in the Lung

The term *aerosol* refers to a collection of small particles that remains airborne for a substantial amount of time. Many pollutants exist in this form, and their pattern of deposition in the lung depends chiefly on their size. The properties of aerosols are also important in understanding the fate of inhaled bronchodilators. Three mechanisms of deposition are recognized.

Impaction

Impaction refers to the tendency of the largest inspired particles to fail to turn the corners of the respiratory tract. As a result, many particles impinge on the mucous surfaces of the nose and pharynx **(Figure 7.2A)** and also on the bifurcations of the large airways. Once a particle strikes a wet surface, it is trapped and not subsequently released. The nose is remarkably efficient at removing the largest particles by this mechanism; almost all particles greater than 20 μm in diameter and approximately 95% of particles 5 μm in diameter are filtered by the nose during resting breathing. **Figure 7.3** shows that most of the deposition of particles over 3 μm in diameter occurs in the nasopharynx during nose breathing.

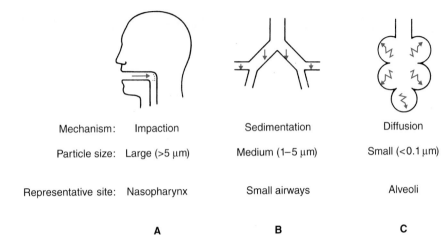

Mechanism:	Impaction	Sedimentation	Diffusion
Particle size:	Large (>5 μm)	Medium (1–5 μm)	Small (<0.1 μm)
Representative site:	Nasopharynx	Small airways	Alveoli
	A	B	C

Figure 7.2. **Scheme of deposition of aerosols in the lung.** The term *representative sites* does not mean that these are the only sites where this form of deposition occurs. For example, impaction also occurs in the medium-sized bronchi, and diffusion also occurs in the large and small airways. (See text for details.)

Sedimentation

Sedimentation is the gradual settling of particles because of their weight **(Figure 7.2B)**. It is particularly important for medium-sized particles (1 to 5 μm) because the larger particles are removed by impaction and the smaller particles settle so slowly. Deposition by sedimentation occurs extensively in

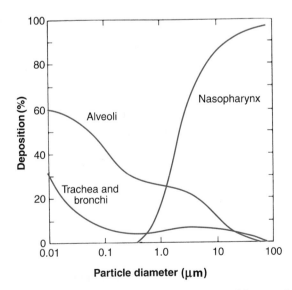

Figure 7.3. **Site of deposition of aerosols.** The largest particles remain in the nasopharynx, but some of the small particles can penetrate to the alveoli.

the small airways, including the terminal and respiratory bronchioles. The chief reason is simply that the dimensions of those airways are small and therefore the particles have a shorter distance to fall. Note that the particles, unlike gases, are not able to diffuse from the respiratory bronchioles to the alveoli because of their negligibly small diffusion rate (see *West's Respiratory Physiology: The Essentials*. 10th ed. p. 7).

Figure 7.4 shows accumulations of dust around the terminal and respiratory bronchioles of a coal miner with early pneumoconiosis. Although the

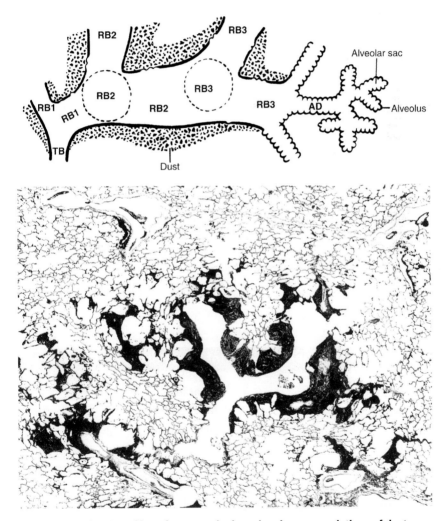

Figure 7.4. Section of lung from a coal miner showing accumulations of dust around the respiratory bronchioles. These small airways show some dilatation, sometimes called focal emphysema. (From Heppleston AG, Leopold JG. Chronic pulmonary emphysema: Anatomy and pathogenesis. *Am J Med* 1961;31:279–291.)

retention of dust depends on both deposition and clearance, and it is possible that some of this dust was transported from peripheral alveoli, the appearance is a graphic reminder of the vulnerability of this region of the lung. It has been suggested that some of the earliest changes in chronic bronchitis and emphysema are secondary to the deposition of atmospheric pollutants (including tobacco smoke particles) in these small airways.

Diffusion

Diffusion is the random movement of particles as a result of their continuous bombardment by gas molecules (**Figure 7.2C**). It occurs to a significant extent only in the smallest particles (less than 0.1 μm in diameter). Deposition by diffusion chiefly takes place in the small airways and alveoli where the distances to the wall are least. However, some deposition by this mechanism also occurs in the larger airways.

Many inhaled particles are not deposited at all but are exhaled with the next breath. In fact, only some 30% of 0.5 μm particles may be left in the lung during normal resting breathing. These particles are too small to impact or sediment to a large extent. In addition, they are too large to diffuse significantly. As a result, they do not move from the terminal and respiratory bronchioles to the alveoli by diffusion, which is the normal mode of gas movement in this region. Small particles may become larger during inspiration by aggregation or by absorbing water.

The pattern of ventilation affects the amount of aerosol deposition. Slow, deep breaths increase the penetration into the lung and thus increase the amount of dust deposited by sedimentation and diffusion. Exercise results in higher rates of airflow and it particularly increases deposition by impaction. In general, deposition of dust is proportional to the ventilation during exercise, which is therefore an important factor during work at the coalface, for example.

Deposition and Clearance of Inhaled Particles

Deposition	Clearance
Impaction	Mucociliary system
Sedimentation	Alveolar macrophages
Diffusion	

Clearance of Deposited Particles

Fortunately, the lung is efficient at removing particles that are deposited within it. Two distinct clearance mechanisms exist: the mucociliary system and the alveolar macrophages (**Figure 7.5**).

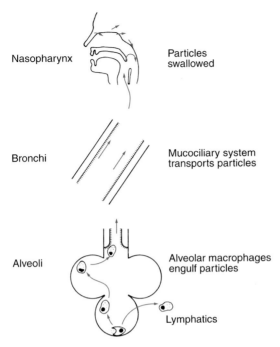

Figure 7.5. Clearance of inhaled particles from the lung. Particles that deposit on the surface of the airways are transported by the mucociliary escalator and swallowed. Particles that reach the alveoli are engulfed by macrophages, which either migrate to the ciliary surface or escape via the lymphatics.

Mucociliary System

Mucus is produced by two sources:

1. Bronchial seromucous glands situated deep in the bronchial walls (see Figures 4.6, 4.7, and 7.6). Both mucus-producing and serous-producing cells are present, and ducts lead the mucus to the airway surface.
2. Goblet cells, which form part of the bronchial epithelium.

The normal mucus film is approximately 5- to 10-μm thick and has two layers **(Figure 7.6)**. The superficial gel layer is relatively tenacious and viscous. As a result, it is efficient at trapping deposited particles. The deeper sol layer is less viscous and thus allows the cilia to beat within it easily. It is likely that the abnormal retention of secretions that occurs in some diseases is caused by changes in the composition of the mucus, with the result that it cannot be propelled easily by the cilia. This occurs in cystic fibrosis and asthma.

The mucus contains the immunoglobulin IgA, which is derived from plasma cells and lymphoid tissue. This humoral factor is an important defense against foreign proteins, bacteria, and viruses.

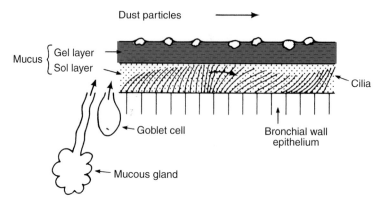

Figure 7.6. Mucociliary escalator. The mucous film consists of a superficial gel layer that traps inhaled particles and a deeper sol layer. It is propelled by cilia.

The cilia are 5- to 7-μm long and beat in a synchronized fashion at between 1,000 and 1,500 times per minute. During the forward stroke, the tips of the cilia apparently come in contact with the gel layer, thus propelling it. However, during the recovery phase, the cilia are bent so much that they move entirely within the sol layer, where the resistance is less.

The mucous blanket moves up at around 1 mm/min in small peripheral airways but as fast as 2 cm/min in the trachea, and eventually, the particles reach the level of the pharynx where they are swallowed. The clearance of a healthy bronchial mucosa is essentially complete in less than 24 hours. In very dusty environments, mucous secretion may be increased so much that cough and expectoration assist in the clearance.

The normal operation of the mucociliary system is affected by pollution and disease. The cilia apparently can be paralyzed by the inhalation of toxic gases, such as oxides of sulfur and nitrogen, and perhaps by tobacco smoke. In acute inflammation of the respiratory tract, as, for example, following influenza infection, the bronchial epithelium may be denuded. Changes in the character of the mucus may occur with infection, thus making it difficult for the cilia to transport it. Mucous plugging of bronchi occurs in asthma, but the mechanism is unknown. Finally, in chronic infections such as bronchiectasis and chronic bronchitis, the volume of secretions may be so great that the ciliary transport system is overwhelmed.

Alveolar Macrophages

The mucociliary system stops short of the alveoli, and particles deposited there are engulfed by macrophages. These amoeboid cells roam around the surface of the alveoli. When they phagocytose foreign particles, either they migrate to the small airways where they load onto the mucociliary escalator (Figure 7.5) or they leave the lung in the lymphatics or possibly the blood. When the dust burden is large or the dust particles are toxic, some of the macrophages migrate through the walls of the respiratory bronchioles and dump their dust there. Figure 7.4 shows the accumulations of dust around the respiratory bronchioles in the lung of a coal miner. If the dust is toxic, such as silica, a fibrous reaction is stimulated in this region.

The macrophages not only transport bacteria out of the lung but also kill them in situ by means of the lysozymes they contain. As a consequence, the alveoli quickly become sterile, although it takes some time for the dead organisms to be cleared from the lung. Immunologic mechanisms are also important in the antibacterial action of macrophages.

Normal macrophage activity can be impaired by various factors, such as cigarette smoke, oxidant gases such as ozone, alveolar hypoxia, radiation, the administration of corticosteroids, and the ingestion of alcohol. Macrophages that engulf particles of silica are often destroyed by this toxic material.

Coal Workers' Pneumoconiosis

The term *pneumoconiosis* refers to parenchymal lung disease caused by inorganic dust inhalation. One form seen in coal workers is directly related to the amount of coal dust to which the miner has been exposed.

Pathology
Early and late forms of the disease should be distinguished. In simple pneumoconiosis, there are aggregations of coal particles around terminal and respiratory bronchioles, with some dilatation of these small airways (Figure 7.4). In the advanced form, known as progressive massive fibrosis, condensed masses of black fibrous tissue infiltrated with dust are seen. Only a small fraction of miners exposed to heavy dust concentrations develop progressive massive fibrosis.

Clinical Features
Simple coal workers' pneumoconiosis apparently causes little disability despite its radiographic appearances. The dyspnea and cough that often accompany the disease are closely related to the smoking history of the miner and are probably chiefly caused by associated chronic bronchitis and emphysema. By contrast, progressive massive fibrosis usually causes increasing dyspnea and may terminate in respiratory failure.

The chest radiograph of simple pneumoconiosis shows a delicate micronodular mottling, and various stages in the advance of the disease are recognized depending on the density of the shadows. Progressive massive fibrosis results in large, irregular dense opacities often surrounded by abnormally radiolucent lung.

Pulmonary Function
Simple pneumoconiosis usually causes little functional impairment by itself. However, sometimes, a small reduction in forced expiratory volume, a rise

in residual volume, and a fall in arterial P_{O_2} are seen. It is often difficult to know whether these changes are caused by associated chronic bronchitis and emphysema.

Progressive massive fibrosis causes a mixed obstructive and restrictive pattern. Distortion of the airways results in irreversible obstructive changes, whereas the large masses of fibrous tissue reduce the useful volume of the lung. Increasing hypoxemia, cor pulmonale, and terminal respiratory failure may occur.

Silicosis

This pneumoconiosis is caused by the inhalation of silica (SiO_2) during quarrying, mining, or sandblasting. Whereas coal dust is virtually inert, silica particles are toxic and provoke a severe fibrous reaction in the lung.

Pathology
Silicotic nodules composed of concentric whorls of dense collagen fibers are found around respiratory bronchioles, inside alveoli, and along the lymphatics. Silica particles may be seen in the nodules.

Clinical Features
Mild forms of the disease may cause no symptoms, although the chest radiograph shows fine nodular markings. Advanced disease results in cough and severe dyspnea, especially on exercise. The radiograph sometimes shows streaks of fibrous tissue, and progressive massive fibrosis may develop. The disease may progress long after exposure to the dust has ceased. There is an increased risk of pulmonary tuberculosis (TB).

Pulmonary Function
The changes are similar to those seen in coal workers' pneumoconiosis but are often more severe. In advanced disease, generalized interstitial fibrosis may develop, with a restrictive type of defect, severe dyspnea and hypoxemia on exercise, and a reduced diffusing capacity.

Asbestos-Related Diseases

Asbestos is a naturally occurring fibrous mineral silicate that is used in a variety of industrial applications, including heat insulation, pipe lagging, roofing materials, and brake linings. Asbestos fibers are long and thin, and it is possible that their aerodynamic characteristics allow them to penetrate far into the lung. When they are in the lung, they may become encased in proteinaceous material. If these are coughed up in the sputum, they are known as asbestos bodies.

Three health hazards are recognized:

1. Diffuse interstitial fibrosis (asbestosis) may gradually occur after heavy exposure. There is a progressive dyspnea (especially on exercise), weakness, and finger clubbing. On auscultation, there are fine basal crepitations. The chest radiograph shows basilar reticular opacities and may show calcified asbestos plaques. Pulmonary function tests in advanced disease reveal a typical restrictive pattern with reductions of vital capacity and lung compliance. A fall in diffusing capacity occurs relatively early in the disease.
2. Bronchial carcinoma is a common complication and the risk is greatly increased by concurrent cigarette smoking.
3. Pleural disease may occur after trivial exposure, for example, in a person who washes the clothes of an asbestos worker. Pleural thickening and plaques are common but are usually harmless. Malignant mesothelioma may develop as much as 40 years after exposure. It causes progressive restriction of chest movement, severe chest pain, and a rapid downhill course and is generally not very amenable to therapy.

Other Pneumoconioses

A variety of other dusts cause simple pneumoconiosis. Examples include iron and its oxides, which cause siderosis and result in a striking, mottled radiographic appearance. Antimony and tin are other culprits. Beryllium exposure results in granulomatous lesions of acute or chronic types. The latter results in interstitial fibrosis with its typical restrictive pattern of dysfunction. The disease is now much less common than it was as a result of strict control of beryllium in industry.

Byssinosis

Some inhaled organic dusts cause airway reactions rather than alveolar reactions. A good example is byssinosis, which follows exposure to cotton dust, especially in the cardroom where the fibers are initially processed.

The pathogenesis is not fully understood, but it appears that the inhalation of some active component in the bracts (leaves around the stem of the cotton boll) leads to the release of histamine from mast cells in the lung. The resulting bronchoconstriction causes dyspnea and wheezing. A feature of the disease is that the symptoms are worse on entering the mill, especially after a period of absence. For this reason, it is sometimes known as "Monday fever." The symptoms include dyspnea, tightness of the chest, wheezing, and an irritating cough. Workers who have already had chronic bronchitis or asthma are especially susceptible.

Pulmonary function tests show an obstructive pattern with reductions in FEV_1, FEV/FVC, $FEF_{25-75\%}$, and FVC. Airway resistance is increased and the amount of inequality of ventilation rises after exposure. Typically, these abnormalities gradually become worse over the course of the working day, but partial or complete recovery occurs during the night or over the weekend. There is no evidence of parenchymal involvement, and the chest radiograph is normal. However, epidemiologic studies show that daily exposure over 20 years or so causes permanent impairment of lung function of the type associated with COPD.

Occupational Asthma

Various occupations involve exposure to allergenic organic dusts, and some individuals develop hypersensitivity. These individuals include flour mill workers who are sensitive to the wheat weevil, lumbar industry workers exposed to western red cedar, printers exposed to gum acacia, and workers handling fur or feathers. Toluene diisocyanate (TDI) is a special case because some individuals develop an extreme sensitivity to this substance, which is used in the manufacture of polyurethane products.

NEOPLASTIC DISEASES

Bronchial Carcinoma

This book is about the function of the diseased lung and how this is measured using pulmonary function tests. For neoplastic diseases, this is generally not an important topic because the effects on pulmonary function are minor in the context of diagnosis, staging, and treatment. In general, the physician's objective is to diagnose the carcinoma early enough to remove it surgically. Pulmonary function tests are only used in this situation to determine whether the patient can tolerate the surgical procedure and are not used for diagnosis. However, lung function is often impaired in moderately advanced disease where surgical removal is usually not an option. Accordingly, this section is relatively brief, and textbooks of pathology or internal medicine should be consulted for additional details on diagnosis, staging, and management of this disease.

Despite being a largely preventable disease, lung cancer continues to have a very high incidence and is now the leading cause of cancer mortality in both men and women in the United States.

Pathogenesis

There is overwhelming evidence that cigarette smoking is a major factor. Epidemiologic studies show that an individual who smokes 20 cigarettes a day has about 20 times the chance of dying from the disease than a nonsmoker of the same age and sex. Furthermore, the risk decreases dramatically if the individual stops smoking.

The specific causative agents in cigarette smoke are uncertain, but many potential carcinogenic substances are present, including aromatic hydrocarbons, phenols, and radioisotopes. Many smoke particles are submicronic and penetrate far into the lung. However, the fact that many bronchogenic carcinomas originate in the large bronchi suggests that deposition by impaction or sedimentation may play an important role (Figure 7.2). Also, the large bronchi are exposed to a high concentration of tobacco smoke products as the material is transported from the more peripheral regions by the mucociliary system. Individuals who inhale other peoples' smoke (passive smokers) also have an increased risk.

Other etiological factors are recognized. Urban dwellers are more at risk, suggesting that atmospheric pollution plays a part. This finding is hardly surprising in view of the variety of chronic respiratory tract irritants that exist in city air (Figure 7.1). Occupational factors also exist, especially exposure to chromates, nickel, arsenic, asbestos, and radioactive gases.

Classification

Most pulmonary neoplasms can be divided into small cell and non–small cell types.

A. *Small cell carcinomas.* These contain a homogeneous population of oat-like cells giving a characteristic appearance. They are highly malignant and have often metastasized by the time of diagnosis. These tumors are seldom seen in peripheral lung and usually do not cavitate.
B. *Non–small cell carcinomas.* This is now the most common form of lung cancer. There are three main types.

   1. *Adenocarcinomas* are now the most common non–small cell carcinoma, with an increasing incidence, particularly among women. They typically occur in the periphery of the lung, show glandular differentiation, and often produce mucus.
   2. *Squamous carcinomas* have a characteristic microscopic appearance in which intercellular bridges are visible, keratin is present, and the cells often form a whorl or nest pattern. Most squamous cell cancers arise in the proximal airways, but peripheral lesions can be seen. Cavitation occurs sometimes with either central or peripheral lesions.
   3. *Large cell carcinomas* are epithelial cancers that lack glandular or squamous features and thus cannot be classified as adenocarcinomas or squamous cell carcinomas. They tend to occur in the periphery of the lung and often demonstrate necrosis.

Bronchioalveolar carcinoma was a term formally used to describe a fourth type of non–small cell carcinoma marked by peripheral location, well-differentiated cytology, growth along alveolar septa, and the ability to spread via the airways or lymphatics. More recent classification schemes now place these tumors in one of several subcategories of adenocarcinoma such as adenocarcinoma in situ or minimally invasive adenocarcinoma.

Many tumors show some heterogeneity of cell type, thus making classification difficult. Also, there are a number of other neoplastic diseases of the respiratory system such as carcinoid tumors or mesothelioma.

Clinical Features
An unproductive cough or hemoptysis is a common early symptom. Sometimes, hoarseness is the first clue and is caused by involvement of the left recurrent laryngeal nerve. Dyspnea caused by pleural effusion or bronchial obstruction and chest pain caused by pleural involvement usually are late symptoms. Examination of the chest is often negative, although signs of lobar collapse or consolidation may be found. The chest radiograph is useful for diagnosis, but small carcinomas may only be visible on CT scan of the chest. CT-guided biopsies and a variety of bronchoscopic techniques are used to facilitate early diagnosis. Sputum cytology may be useful in a limited number of patients.

Pulmonary Function
As stated earlier, the physician's objective is to diagnose a carcinoma of the bronchus early enough to remove it surgically. While lung function is typically normal in early disease, it is often impaired in moderately advanced severe disease. A large pleural effusion causes a restrictive defect, as may the collapse of a lobe after complete bronchial obstruction. Partial obstruction of a large bronchus can result in an obstructive pattern. The obstruction can be caused either by a tumor of the bronchial wall or by compression by an enlarged lymph gland. Sometimes, the movement of the lung on the affected side is seen to lag behind the normal lung, and air may cycle back and forth between the normal and obstructed lobes (see *West's Respiratory Physiology: The Essentials*. 10th ed. p. 191). This cycle is known as pendelluft (swinging air). Complete obstruction of a mainstem bronchus can give a pseudorestrictive pattern because half of the lung is not ventilating. Partial or complete bronchial obstruction usually causes some hypoxemia.

INFECTIOUS DISEASES

Infectious diseases are of great importance in pulmonary medicine. However, they generally do not cause specific patterns of impaired pulmonary function, and pulmonary function tests are of little value in the evaluation of these patients. Since this book is about the function of the diseased lung and its measurement using pulmonary function tests, infectious diseases do not merit much prominence. A textbook on internal medicine or pathology should be consulted for further details.

Pneumonia

This term refers to inflammation of the lung parenchyma associated with alveolar filling by exudate.

Pathology

The alveoli are crammed with cells, chiefly polymorphonuclear leukocytes. Resolution often occurs with restoration of the normal morphology. However, suppuration may result in necrosis of tissue, causing a lung abscess. Special forms of pneumonia include that following aspiration of gastric fluid or oral secretions or animal or mineral oil (lipoid pneumonia).

Clinical Features

These features vary considerably depending on the causative organism, the age of the patient, and his or her general condition. The usual features include malaise, fever, and cough, which is often productive of purulent sputum. Pleuritic pain is common and is worse on deep breathing. Examination reveals rapid shallow breathing, tachycardia, and sometimes cyanosis. Often, there are signs of consolidation, and the chest radiograph shows opacification (**Figure 7.7**). This may involve all of a lobe (lobar pneumonia), but frequently, the distribution is

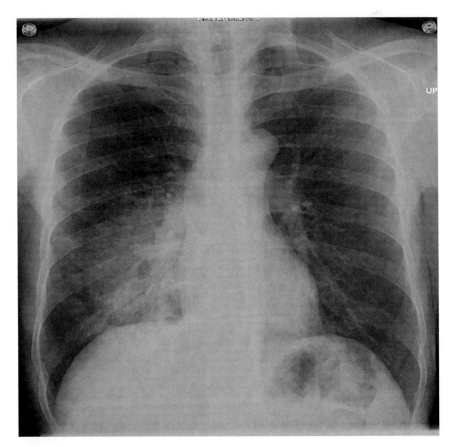

Figure 7.7. Chest radiograph from a patient with pneumonia. There is an opacity in the right lower lobe.

patchy (bronchopneumonia). Sputum examination and culture frequently identify the causative organism, although some common causes of pneumonia, such as *Legionella* and mycoplasma, do not readily grow on routine culture media.

Pulmonary Function

Because the pneumonic region is not ventilated, it causes shunt and hypoxemia. The severity of these conditions depends on the amount of lung affected by the pneumonia and the local pulmonary blood flow, which may be substantially reduced either by the disease process itself or by hypoxic vasoconstriction. While patients with severe pneumonia may be cyanosed, carbon dioxide retention does not generally occur. Chest movement may be restricted by pleural pain or by a pleural effusion.

Tuberculosis

Pulmonary TB takes many forms. Advanced disease is much less common now in many parts of the world because of improvements in public health and increasing availability of effective antituberculous drugs, although the disease remains common in places like sub-Saharan Africa, particularly among people infected with human immunodeficiency virus (HIV).

Upon initial infection, referred to as primary TB, the majority of people remain asymptomatic, although some develop fever, parenchymal opacities, and hilar lymphadenopathy. Isolated pleural effusions may also be seen. Whether or not patients manifest symptoms, once the primary infection is controlled, bacilli often remain in the patient, contained within granulomas. This situation, referred to as latent TB infection, can be identified by a hypersensitivity response on TB skin testing or through assays that detect interferon gamma release from blood lymphocytes stimulated by TB antigens.

If cell-mediated immunity is preserved, most patients never develop active disease again. Individuals who have defects in cell-mediated immunity through, for example, HIV infection or use of immunosuppressive medications can develop reactivation TB, which often presents with subacute onset of dyspnea, productive cough, hemoptysis, and constitutional symptoms along with upper lobe opacities, fibrosis, and cavitation. Extensive fibrosis can lead to restrictive impairments in pulmonary function.

While effective treatments for TB are readily available, cases are still seen in high-income countries due to the increasing ease of travel and frequency of immigration from TB-endemic regions. The emergence of multidrug and extremely drug-resistant strains of the bacillus (MDR-TB and XDR-TB, respectively) remains on ongoing concern.

Fungus Infections

Fungi cause several pulmonary diseases, including *Histoplasmosis*, *Coccidiomycosis*, and *Blastomycosis*. Because the organisms are endemic to particular regions of the country, infection is generally only seen in individuals who live in or travel to regions associated with these organisms, such as the San Joaquin Valley in California or other areas of the southwestern United States where *Coccidiomycosis* is seen. Many infections are asymptomatic, while severe disease may be seen with large exposure or in immunocompromised individuals. *Cryptococcus* species can also cause pneumonia in both immunocompetent and immunosuppressed individuals.

Pulmonary Involvement in HIV

HIV frequently involves the lung, with the risk and type of infection being a function of the degree of immunosuppression. Bacterial pneumonia and TB may occur with any degree of immunosuppression, while infections such as *Pneumocystis jirovecii*, *Mycobacterium avium–intracellulare*, and cytomegalovirus infections occur when the CD4+ count falls below certain thresholds. Kaposi's sarcoma may occur in the lung. When patients from high-risk groups, such as injection drug users or people who have promiscuous unprotected intercourse, present with these pulmonary problems, they should be evaluated for HIV.

SUPPURATIVE DISEASES

Bronchiectasis

This disease is characterized by permanent dilatation of bronchi with local suppuration, as a result of chronic infection and inflammation and, in some cases, impaired airway clearance. It is seen in conjunction with a variety of problems such as recurrent pneumonia, underlying immunodeficiencies such as hypogammaglobulinemia, ciliary dyskinesias, or airway occlusion due to, for example, a retained airway foreign body or chronic extrinsic compression.

Pathology
The mucosal surface of the affected bronchi shows loss of ciliated epithelium, squamous metaplasia, and infiltration with inflammatory cells. Pus is present in the lumen during infective exacerbations. In advanced stages, the surrounding lung often shows fibrosis and chronic inflammatory changes.

Clinical Features
The cardinal feature is a chronic productive cough with copious amounts of yellow or green sputum that can be exacerbated following upper respiratory tract infections. Patients may have halitosis and are prone to massive hemoptysis due to hypertrophy of the bronchial circulation. Crepitations are often heard, and finger clubbing is seen in severe cases. The chest radiograph shows increased parenchymal markings and dilated airways with thickened walls. Dilated airways are readily seen on CT scans of the chest (**Figure 7.8**).

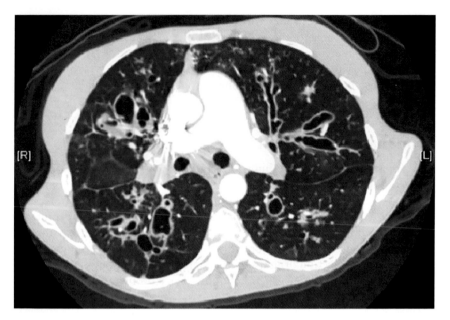

Figure 7.8. CT scan of the chest demonstrating dilated, thickened airways in a patient with bronchiectasis due to cystic fibrosis.

Pulmonary Function

Mild disease causes no loss of function. In more advanced cases, there is a reduction of FEV_1 and FVC because of chronic inflammatory changes, including fibrosis. Radioactive isotope measurements show reduced ventilation and pulmonary blood flow in the affected area, but there may be a greatly increased bronchial artery supply to the diseased tissue. Hypoxemia may develop as a result of blood flow through unventilated lung.

Cystic Fibrosis

Cystic fibrosis is caused by the loss of function of the cystic fibrosis transmembrane regulator (CFTR), a transmembrane protein present in a variety of cell types and tissues. While the lung is the primary affected organ, CF also affects the liver, pancreas, gonads, and other organs.

Pathology

A large number of mutations affect the CFTR through a variety of mechanisms such as absent or deficient production of the protein, abnormal protein folding, or abnormal transport to the cell membrane. The net result of all of these defects are varying degrees of impaired sodium and chloride transport, which lead to impaired mucous clearance or plugging of airways or ducts. In the lungs, decreased sodium efflux from the respiratory epithelium reduces hydration of the periciliary mucous layer, and this impairs mucociliary clearance and predisposes to infection.

Atrophy of pancreatic tissue and dilatation of pancreatic ducts can occur, leading to both exocrine and endocrine insufficiency. The first impairs absorption of fat soluble vitamins causing malnutrition, while the second leads to diabetes mellitus. Thickened secretions and chronic inflammation in the bile ductules can lead to portal hypertension and cirrhosis. The majority of male patients are infertile due to obstructive azoospermia from absence or atrophy of male reproductive tract structures.

Clinical Features

Some patients present with features of the disease at birth or early in life such as meconium ileus, recurrent infections, or failure to thrive. Less severe presentations might not occur until later in childhood or even adulthood. The respiratory symptoms include cough productive of copious thick sputum, frequent chest infections, and decreased exercise tolerance. Some patients cough up blood, which comes from bronchiectatic areas. Finger clubbing is often prominent. Auscultation may reveal coarse rales and rhonchi. The chest radiograph is abnormal early in the disease and shows areas of consolidation, fibrosis, and cystic changes. Many cases are now detected from elevated serum immunoreactive trypsinogen during neonatal screening. Diagnosis is confirmed by finding elevated sweat chloride levels, specific gene mutations, or an abnormal nasal potential difference.

For many years, death almost invariably occurred before adulthood, but with improved treatment focused on secretion clearance, suppressive antibiotic therapy, and aggressive treatment of exacerbations, the median survival is now greater than 40 years of age.

Pulmonary Function

An abnormal distribution of ventilation and an increased alveolar–arterial O_2 difference are early changes. Some investigators report that tests of small airway function, such as flow rates at low lung volumes, may detect minimal disease. There are decreases in FEV_1 and $FEF_{25-75\%}$ that do not respond to bronchodilators. RV and FRC are raised and there may be loss of elastic recoil. Exercise tolerance falls as the disease progresses, and in later stages, patients often manifest a mixed obstructive–restrictive defect on pulmonary function testing.

KEY CONCEPTS

1. The most important atmospheric pollutants include carbon monoxide, oxides of nitrogen and sulfur, hydrocarbons, particulates, and photochemical oxidants.

2. Most pollutants occur as aerosols and are deposited in the lung by impaction, sedimentation, or diffusion.

3. Deposited pollutants are removed by the mucociliary system in the airways and macrophages in the alveoli.

4. Coal workers' pneumoconiosis results from long-term exposure to coal dust. In its mild form, it causes dyspnea and cough together with mottling of the chest radiograph, but sometimes, the role of chronic bronchitis in the symptoms is difficult to differentiate in a smoker.

5. Other pneumoconioses include asbestos-related diseases. Byssinosis is caused by organic cotton dust. Occupational asthma also occurs in some industries.

6. Infectious diseases of the lung including bacterial pneumonia, fungal infections, and TB are an important source of morbidity and mortality in high- and low-income countries but generally do not require pulmonary function tests.

7. Bronchial carcinoma is largely caused by cigarette smoking and is the most common cause of cancer-related death in the United States. The prognosis varies based on the type and stage of the cancer.

8. Cystic fibrosis is a genetic abnormality of the CFTR, which causes abnormal mucus, bronchiectasis, and impaired pulmonary function. Good medical treatment has greatly increased the lifespan of these patients.

CLINICAL VIGNETTE

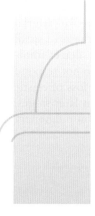

A 19-year-old man presents to the emergency department after coughing up a large amount of blood. During an evaluation by his pediatrician at the age of 5 for recurrent sinus and respiratory infections, he was found to have an elevated sweat chloride test and two gene mutations associated with cystic fibrosis. He was on appropriate treatment for several years, but since dropping out of school and moving out of his parent's house, he has not been taking any medications or doing his regular airway clearance techniques. He states that his breathing has been getting worse over the past 6 months and that he has a daily cough productive of large amounts of thick yellow sputum. On examination, he is afebrile but tachypneic. He has diffuse rhonchi throughout his lungs, a prolonged expiratory phase, and finger clubbing. A chest radiograph is obtained and shows the following:

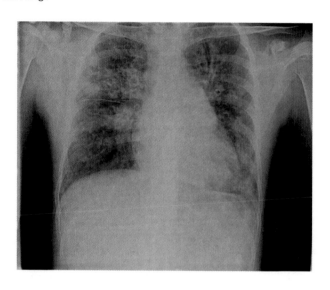

Questions

- What is the pathophysiological basis of his disease?
- What are the tubular structures seen in the mid–upper lung zones on his chest radiograph?
- What changes in pulmonary function would you expect to see on detailed pulmonary function testing?
- Why are regular airway clearance techniques important for the long-term health of this patient?
- Why is he coughing up large amounts of blood?

QUESTIONS

1. Concerning smog:
   A. Ozone is mainly produced in automobile engines.
   B. A temperature inversion occurs when the air near the ground is hotter than the air above.
   C. The main source of sulfur oxides is the automobile.
   D. Nitrogen oxides can cause inflammation of the upper respiratory tract.
   E. Scrubbing flue gases is ineffective in removing particulates.

2. Concerning cigarette smoke:
   A. Inhaled smoke contains negligible amounts of carbon monoxide.
   B. Cigarette smokers can have enough carboxyhemoglobin in their blood to impair mental skills.
   C. Nicotine is not addictive.
   D. The risk of coronary heart disease is not affected by smoking.
   E. The concentration of pollutants in cigarette smoke is less than in the air of a large city on a smoggy day.

3. In a coal miner, the deposition of coal dust in the lung will be reduced by:
   A. Frequent coughing.
   B. Exercise.
   C. Mining operations that produce very small dust particles.
   D. Rapid deep breathing.
   E. Nose breathing, as opposed to mouth breathing.

4. Concerning the mucociliary escalator in the lung:
   A. Most of the mucus comes from goblet cells in the epithelium.
   B. Trapped particles move more slowly in the trachea than in the peripheral airways.
   C. Normal clearances take several days.
   D. The cilia beat about twice a second.
   E. The composition of the mucous film is altered in some diseases.

5. Concerning bronchial carcinoma:
   A. It is a less common cause of death than breast cancer among women in the United States.
   B. The specific carcinogenic agent in cigarette smoke is known.
   C. Pulmonary function tests are important in the early detection of the disease.
   D. Non–small cell carcinomas are the most common type.
   E. A carcinoma is always visible on a good chest radiograph.

6. A 70-year-old man with no smoking history presents with 8 months of worsening dyspnea and a nonproductive cough. He spent many years as an insulation worker in the shipyards. On exam, he has a fast respiratory rate with small volumes and fine crepitations at the bases of his lungs. A plain chest radiograph reveals basilar net-like opacities and calcified pleural plaques. Spirometry shows an FEV_1 of 65% predicted, an FVC of 69% predicted, and FEV_1/FVC ratio of 0.83. Which of the following is the most likely diagnosis?
   A. Asbestosis
   B. Berylliosis
   C. Chronic obstructive pulmonary disease
   D. Coal-worker's pneumoconiosis
   E. Silicosis

7. A 24-year-old woman with a 5-year history of injection drug use but no other past medical history is evaluated for worsening dyspnea and a dry cough over a period of 2 weeks. On exam, she is tachypneic with an oxygen saturation of 85% breathing air. Her neck veins are not elevated, her cardiac exam is normal, and she has diffuse rhonchi on auscultation. After a chest radiograph reveals diffuse bilateral opacities, a sputum sample is obtained and shows evidence of *Pneumocystis jirovecii* pneumonia. Which of the following is the most appropriate next diagnostic test?
   A. Echocardiography
   B. HIV antibody test
   C. Spirometry
   D. Sweat chloride testing
   E. Tuberculosis skin test

8. Following an accident in a paper mill, it is found that the particles released into the air were 20 to 30 μm in diameter. Where in the respiratory tracts of the workers in the plant at the time of the accident were the particles most likely to have deposited?
   A. Alveolar space
   B. Bronchi
   C. Nose and nasopharynx
   D. Respiratory bronchioles
   E. Terminal bronchioles

9. A 46-year-old man is evaluated for 2 days of fever, worsening dyspnea, and cough productive of rust-colored sputum. His oxygen saturation at the time of presentation is 88% breathing air. He is sweating and tachypneic, with dullness to percussion and decreased breath sounds at his right lung base. A chest radiograph demonstrates a focal opacity in the right lower lobe. Which of the following statements regarding this patient's diagnosis is true?
   A. Shunt is the most likely cause of his hypoxemia.
   B. He is likely to have carbon dioxide retention.
   C. Following resolution, he will have a fibrotic scar in his right lung.
   D. All common bacterial causes grow on routine culture media.
   E. Blood flow through the affected area of his lung is increased.

10. Shortly after birth, a baby boy develops meconium ileus and, on further testing, is found to have an elevated sweat chloride level. Which of the following statements best characterize the future issues that will affect this child?
   A. He is unlikely to live past 20 years of age.
   B. He is highly likely to be infertile.
   C. Extrapulmonary involvement is unlikely to occur.
   D. Mucociliary function in the airways will be unaffected.
   E. He will not require treatment once past the age of 5.

PART THREE

FUNCTION OF THE FAILING LUNG

8 ▪ **Respiratory Failure**

9 ▪ **Oxygen Therapy**

10 ▪ **Mechanical Ventilation**

Respiratory failure is the result of many types of acute or chronic lung disease. Part Three is devoted to the physiologic principles of respiratory failure and its chief modes of treatment: oxygen administration and mechanical ventilation.

RESPIRATORY FAILURE

8

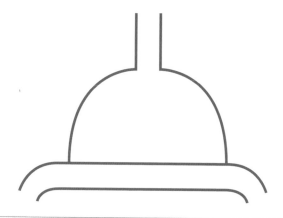

- **Gas Exchange in Respiratory Failure**
  Patterns of Arterial Blood Gases
  Hypoxemia of Respiratory Failure
  Causes
  Detection
  Tissue Hypoxia
  Effects of Severe Hypoxemia
  Hypercapnia in Respiratory Failure
  Causes
  Effects
  Acidosis in Respiratory Failure
  Role of Diaphragm Fatigue

- **Types of Respiratory Failure**
  Acute Overwhelming Lung Disease
  Neuromuscular Disorders
  Acute or Chronic Lung Disease
  Acute Respiratory Distress
  Syndrome
  Pathology
  Pathogenesis
  Clinical Features
  Pulmonary Function

  Infant Respiratory Distress
  Syndrome

- **Management of Respiratory Failure**
  Hypoxemia
  Hypercapnia
  Airway Resistance
  Compliance
  Respiratory Infection
  Cardiac Insufficiency

Respiratory failure is said to occur when the lung fails to oxygenate the arterial blood adequately and/or fails to prevent CO_2 retention. It can be an acute or chronic process. There is no absolute definition of the levels of arterial P_{O_2} and P_{CO_2} that indicate respiratory failure. However, a P_{O_2} of less than 60 mm Hg or a P_{CO_2} of more than 50 mm Hg are numbers that are often quoted. In practice, the significance of such values depends considerably on the patient's history.

GAS EXCHANGE IN RESPIRATORY FAILURE

Patterns of Arterial Blood Gases

Various types of respiratory failure are associated with different degrees of hypoxemia and CO_2 retention. **Figure 8.1** shows an O_2–CO_2 diagram (see *West's Respiratory Physiology: The Essentials.* 10th ed. pp. 187–189) with the line for a respiratory exchange ratio of 0.8. Pure *hypoventilation* leading to respiratory failure moves the arterial P_{O_2} and P_{CO_2} in the direction indicated by arrow A. This pattern occurs in respiratory failure caused by neuromuscular disease, such as Guillain-Barré syndrome, or by an overdose of a narcotic drug (see Figures 2.2 and 2.3). Severe *ventilation–perfusion ratio inequality* with alveolar ventilation inadequate to maintain a normal arterial P_{CO_2} results in movement along a line, such as B. The hypoxemia is more severe in relation to the hypercapnia than in the case of pure hypoventilation. Such a pattern is frequently seen in the respiratory failure of chronic obstructive pulmonary disease (COPD).

Severe interstitial disease sometimes results in movement along line C. Here, there is increasingly severe hypoxemia but no CO_2 retention because of the raised ventilation. This pattern may be seen in advanced diffuse interstitial lung disease or sarcoidosis. Sometimes, there is a rise in arterial P_{CO_2}, but this is typically less marked than in obstructive diseases.

In respiratory failure caused by the acute respiratory distress syndrome (ARDS), the arterial P_{CO_2} may be low, as shown by line D, but the hypox-

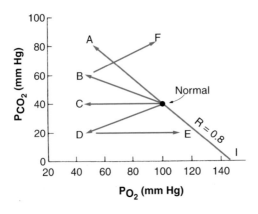

Figure 8.1. Patterns of arterial P_{O_2} and P_{CO_2} in different types of respiratory failure. Note that the P_{CO_2} can be high, as in pure hypoventilation (*line A*), or low, as in ARDS (*line D*). The lines from *B* to *F* and from *D* to *E* show the effects of oxygen breathing. (See text for further details.)

emia may be extreme. Such patients are usually treated with added inspired oxygen, which raises the arterial P_{O_2} but often does not affect the P_{CO_2} (D to E), although in some instances, P_{CO_2} may rise. Oxygen therapy to patients whose respiratory failure is caused by COPD improves the arterial P_{O_2} but frequently causes a rise in P_{CO_2} because of decreased ventilation (B to F) as well as changes in ventilation–perfusion matching due to reduction of hypoxic pulmonary vasoconstriction.

Hypoxemia of Respiratory Failure

Causes
Any of the four mechanisms of hypoxemia—hypoventilation, diffusion impairment, shunt, and ventilation–perfusion inequality—can contribute to the severe hypoxemia of respiratory failure. However, the most important cause by far is ventilation–perfusion inequality (including blood flow through unventilated lung). This mechanism is largely responsible for the low arterial P_{O_2} in respiratory failure complicating obstructive diseases, restrictive diseases, and ARDS.

Detection
While signs such as cyanosis, tachycardia, and altered mental status provide clues to the presence of hypoxemia, most patients are initially identified as being hypoxemic by the presence of a low oxygen saturation on pulse oximetry. Once hypoxemia is identified in this way, measuring the P_{O_2} by arterial blood gas is helpful to determine the degree of hypoxemia and assess the adequacy of ventilation.

Tissue Hypoxia
Hypoxemia is dangerous because it causes tissue hypoxia. However, the arterial P_{O_2} is only one factor in the delivery of oxygen to the tissues. Other factors include the oxygen capacity of the blood, the oxygen affinity of the hemoglobin, cardiac output, and the distribution of blood flow.

Tissues vary considerably in their vulnerability to hypoxia. Those at greatest risk include the central nervous system and the myocardium. Cessation of blood flow to the cerebral cortex results in loss of function within 4 to 6 seconds, loss of consciousness in 10 to 20 seconds, and irreversible changes in 3 to 5 minutes.

If the tissue P_{O_2} falls below a critical level, aerobic oxidation ceases, and anaerobic glycolysis takes over with the formation and release of increasing amounts of lactic acid. The P_{O_2} at which this occurs is not accurately known and probably varies among tissues. However, there is evidence that the critical intracellular P_{O_2} is of the order of 1 to 3 mm Hg in the region of the mitochondria.

Anaerobic glycolysis is a relatively inefficient method of obtaining energy from glucose. Nevertheless, it plays a critical role in maintaining tissue viability in respiratory failure. Large amounts of lactic acid are formed and released into the blood, causing a metabolic acidosis. If tissue oxygenation subsequently improves, the lactic acid can be reconverted to glucose or used directly for energy. Most of this reconversion takes place in the liver.

Effects of Severe Hypoxemia

Mild hypoxemia produces few physiologic changes. It should be recalled that the arterial oxygen saturation is still approximately 90% when the P_{O_2} is only 60 mm Hg at a normal pH (see Figure 2.1). The only abnormalities are a slight impairment of mental performance, diminished visual acuity, and perhaps mild hyperventilation.

When the arterial P_{O_2} drops quickly below 40 to 50 mm Hg, deleterious effects are seen in several organ systems. The central nervous system is particularly vulnerable, and the patient often has headache, somnolence, or clouding of consciousness. Profound acute hypoxemia may cause convulsions, retinal hemorrhages, and permanent brain damage. Tachycardia and mild hypertension are often seen, partly due to the release of catecholamines, but in severe cases, patients can develop bradycardia and hypotension and even go into cardiac arrest. Renal function is impaired, and sodium retention and proteinuria may be seen. Pulmonary hypertension can also be seen because of associated alveolar hypoxia and hypoxic pulmonary vasoconstriction.

Hypercapnia in Respiratory Failure

Causes

Both mechanisms of CO_2 retention—hypoventilation and ventilation–perfusion inequality—can be important in respiratory failure. Hypoventilation is the cause in respiratory failure resulting from neuromuscular diseases such as amyotrophic lateral sclerosis and Guillain-Barré syndrome, narcotic drug overdose, or a chest wall abnormality such as severe kyphoscoliosis (see Figure 2.3 and Table 2.1). Ventilation–perfusion inequality is the culprit in severe COPD and long-standing interstitial disease.

An important cause of CO_2 retention in select patients with respiratory failure is the injudicious use of oxygen therapy. Many patients with severe COPD gradually develop severe hypoxemia and some CO_2 retention over a period of months. These patients are often referred to as having chronic respiratory failure and can live in this state for long periods. However, such a patient usually has a high work of breathing (see Figure 4.13), and much of the ventilatory drive comes from hypoxic stimulation of the peripheral chemoreceptors. The arterial pH is nearly normal because of renal retention of bicarbonate (compensated respiratory acidosis), and the pH of the cerebrospinal fluid (CSF) is also nearly normal because of an increase in bicarbonate there. Thus, despite an increased arterial P_{CO_2}, the main ventilatory drive comes from the hypoxemia.

If this patient develops a relatively mild intercurrent respiratory infection and is treated with a high inspired oxygen concentration, a dangerous situation can rapidly develop. The hypoxic ventilatory drive may be abolished while the work of breathing is increased because of retained secretions or bronchospasm. As a result, the ventilation may become grossly depressed and high levels of arterial P_{CO_2} may develop. In addition, profound hypoxemia may ensue if the oxygen is discontinued. This is because even if the ventilation does return to its previous level, the patient may take many minutes to unload the large accumulation of CO_2 in the tissues because of the large body stores of this gas.

Another cause of CO_2 retention in these patients is the release of hypoxic vasoconstriction in poorly ventilated areas of lung as a result of the increased alveolar P_{O_2}. The consequences of this are increased blood flow to $\dot{V}_A/\dot{Q}$ low areas and worsening of inequality that exaggerates the CO_2 retention. This factor is probably less important than the depression of ventilation, but the rapidity of the rise in arterial P_{CO_2} when some of these patients are given oxygen suggests that this mechanism may play a part.

In addition to patients with severe COPD, this phenomenon can also be seen in morbidly obese patients with obesity hypoventilation syndrome.

These groups of patients present a therapeutic dilemma. While oxygen administration is necessary to relieve potentially life-threatening hypoxemia, it may also cause severe CO_2 retention and respiratory acidosis. The answer to this problem is to give just enough oxygen to raise the oxygen saturation to 88–94% and to monitor the arterial blood gases frequently to determine whether the respiratory acidosis is worsening. The use of added oxygen is discussed further in Chapter 9.

Effects

Raised levels of P_{CO_2} in the blood greatly increase cerebral blood flow, causing headache, raised CSF pressure, and sometimes, papilledema. In practice, the cerebral effects of hypercapnia overlap with the effects of hypoxemia. The resulting abnormalities include restlessness, tremor, slurred speech, asterixis (flapping tremor), and fluctuations of mood. High levels of P_{CO_2} are narcotic and cloud consciousness, particularly when they develop acutely.

Acidosis in Respiratory Failure

The CO_2 retention causes a respiratory acidosis that may be severe. However, patients who gradually develop respiratory failure may retain considerable amounts of bicarbonate, keeping the fall of pH in check (see Figure 2.10). However, acute exacerbations of their underlying disease can further raise their P_{CO_2} and worsen the pH.

Acidemia may also worsen if CO_2 retention is accompanied by severe hypoxemia and tissue hypoxia, which, as noted, can lead to liberation of lactic acid and a metabolic acidosis. This can be exacerbated by factors that impair end-organ perfusion such as shock or decreased venous return due to increased intrathoracic pressure during mechanical ventilation.

Role of Diaphragm Fatigue

Fatigue of the diaphragm can contribute to the hypoventilation of respiratory failure, but its full role is not completely understood. The diaphragm consists of striated skeletal muscle innervated by the phrenic nerves. Although the diaphragm is predominantly made up of slow-twitch oxidative fibers and fast-twitch oxidative glycolytic fibers, which are relatively resistant to fatigue, this can occur if the work of breathing is greatly increased over prolonged periods of time. Fatigue can be defined as a loss of contractile force after work; it can be measured directly from the transdiaphragmatic pressure resulting from a maximum contraction or indirectly from the muscle relaxation time or the electromyogram, although neither technique is commonly used at the bedside.

There is evidence that some patients with severe COPD continually breathe close to the work level at which fatigue occurs and that an exacerbation or infection can tip them into a fatigue state. This will then result in hypoventilation, CO_2 retention, and severe hypoxemia. Because hypercapnia impairs diaphragm contractility and severe hypoxemia accelerates the onset of fatigue, a vicious cycle develops. This situation can be limited by reducing the work of breathing by treating bronchospasm and controlling infection and by giving oxygen judiciously to relieve the hypoxemia. The force of contraction can be improved through pulmonary rehabilitation programs. While the administration of methylxanthines may improve diaphragm contractility and also relieve reversible bronchoconstriction, they are no longer widely used in clinical practice for this purpose.

TYPES OF RESPIRATORY FAILURE

A large number of conditions can lead to respiratory failure, and various classifications are possible. However, from the point of view of the physiological principles of management, five groups can be distinguished:

1. Acute overwhelming lung disease
2. Neuromuscular disorders
3. Acute or chronic lung disease
4. ARDS
5. Infant respiratory distress syndrome

Acute Overwhelming Lung Disease

Many acute diseases, if severe enough, can lead to respiratory failure. These include infections such as fulminating viral or bacterial pneumonias, vascular diseases such as pulmonary embolism, and exposure to inhaled toxic substances such as chlorine gas or oxides of nitrogen. Respiratory failure supervenes as the primary disease progresses, and profound hypoxemia with or without hypercapnia develops. In addition to treating the underlying cause, oxygen administration is required for the hypoxemia, and mechanical ventilation may be necessary to support the patient until they recover. Extracorporeal membrane oxygenators (ECMO) that largely take over the gas exchange function of the lung are being used with increasing frequency in very severe cases refractory to other forms of support. This group of conditions merges into ARDS (see the section "Acute Respiratory Distress Syndrome" later in this chapter).

Neuromuscular Disorders

Respiratory failure may occur when brainstem respiratory centers are depressed by drugs, such as opiates and benzodiazepines. Other conditions include central nervous system and neuromuscular diseases such as encephalitis, poliomyelitis, botulism, Guillain-Barré syndrome, myasthenia gravis, anticholinesterase poisoning, amyotrophic lateral sclerosis, and muscular dystrophy (see Figure 2.3 and Table 2.1). Trauma to the chest wall can also be responsible.

In these conditions, the essential feature is hypoventilation leading to CO_2 retention with moderate hypoxemia (see Figures 2.2 and 8.1). Respiratory acidosis occurs, but the magnitude of the fall in pH depends on the rapidity and duration of the increase in P_{CO_2} and the extent of the renal compensation.

In addition to treating the underlying disease when feasible, invasive mechanical ventilation is often necessary in these conditions, and occasionally, as in bulbar poliomyelitis, it may be required for months or even years. However, the lung itself is often normal, and, if so, little or no additional oxygen is necessary. Noninvasive ventilatory support, in which positive pressure is delivered through a tight-fitting mask rather than an endotracheal tube, is sometimes used in patients with normal mental status and for whom the duration of impairment is expected to be only a few days.

Acute or Chronic Lung Disease

This refers to an acute exacerbation of disease in a patient with long-standing underlying disease. It is an important and common group that includes patients with chronic bronchitis and emphysema, asthma, and cystic fibrosis. Many patients with COPD follow a gradual downhill course with increasingly severe hypoxemia and CO_2 retention over months or years. Such patients are usually capable of limited physical activity even though both the arterial P_{O_2} and P_{CO_2} may be in the region of 50 mm Hg. This situation is often referred to as chronic respiratory failure, as opposed to the acute form seen in problems like pneumonia or pulmonary embolism.

However, if such a patient develops even a mild exacerbation or chest infection, the condition often deteriorates rapidly, with profound hypoxemia, CO_2 retention, and respiratory acidosis. The reserves of pulmonary function are minimal, and any increase in the work of breathing or worsening of ventilation–perfusion relationships as a result of retained secretions or bronchospasm pushes the patient over the brink into frank respiratory failure.

The treatment of these patients is challenging. In addition to treating the underlying problem, supplemental oxygen is necessary to relieve the severe hypoxemia. However, as noted earlier, changes in ventilation–perfusion matching and loss of ventilatory drive can worsen CO_2 retention and acidosis if too much oxygen is administered. For this reason, it is usual to give enough oxygen to raise the oxygen saturation to 88–94% and monitor closely for signs of worsening hypercarbia (see Chapter 9).

Mechanical ventilation may be necessary in many cases. In patients with severe underlying disease, intubation and invasive mechanical ventilation pose a dilemma, as it may be difficult or impossible to wean them from this support. The increasing use of noninvasive ventilation in management of severe COPD exacerbations has alleviated this problem to some extent and improved outcomes for these patients.

Acute Respiratory Distress Syndrome

An important cause of acute respiratory failure, ARDS, is an end result of a variety of insults both intrinsic to the lung, such as pneumonia or aspiration, and extrinsic to the lung including burns, trauma, sepsis from nonpulmonary sources, and pancreatitis.

Pathology

The early changes consist of interstitial and alveolar edema. Hemorrhage, cellular debris, and proteinaceous fluid are present in the alveoli, hyaline membranes may be seen, and there is patchy atelectasis **(Figure 8.2)**. Later, hyperplasia and organization occur. The damaged alveolar epithelium

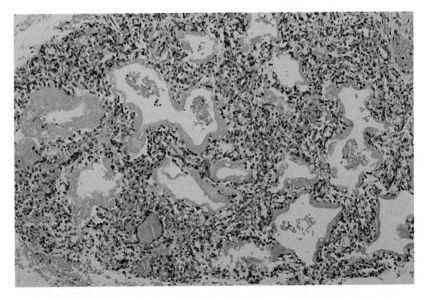

Figure 8.2. Histologic changes in ARDS as found on autopsy. There is patchy atelectasis, edema, hyaline membranes, and hemorrhage in the alveoli as well as inflammatory cells in the alveolar walls. (Image courtesy of Edward Klatt, MD.)

becomes lined with type 2 alveolar epithelial cells, and there is cellular infiltration of the alveolar walls. Eventually, interstitial fibrosis may develop, although complete healing can occur.

Pathogenesis
This is still unclear and many factors play a role. As a result of the initial injury, proinflammatory cytokines including various interleukins and tumor necrosis factor are released, leading to neutrophil recruitment and activation. These neutrophils subsequently release reactive oxygen species, proteases, and cytokines that damage type 1 alveolar epithelial cells and capillary endothelial cells, leading to increased capillary permeability and flooding of the alveoli and interstitium with proteinaceous fluid.

Clinical Features
ARDS may develop anywhere from several hours to 7 days following the initial insult. The onset is typically heralded by worsening hypoxemia and increasing oxygen requirements, at which time the chest radiograph typically shows increasing bilateral alveolar opacities as in **Figure 8.3**. The severity of hypoxemia, which is assessed by measuring the ratio of the Pa_{O_2} to FiO_2, varies

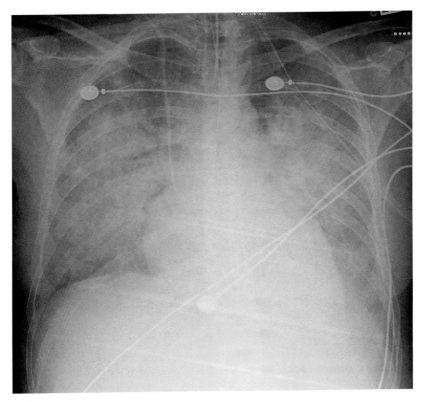

Figure 8.3. Radiograph showing typical changes in ARDS.

> ## Acute Respiratory Distress Syndrome
>
> End result of a variety of insults including trauma and infection
> Hemorrhagic edema with opacification on the radiograph
> Severe hypoxemia
> Low lung compliance
> Mechanical ventilation typically required
> High mortality

significantly between patients. Improvements in ICU care have decreased the mortality related to ARDS to about 20–25% of cases.

Pulmonary Function

The lung becomes very stiff, and unusually high pressures are required to ventilate it mechanically. Associated with this reduced compliance is a marked fall in functional residual capacity (FRC). The cause of the increased recoil is presumably the alveolar edema and exudate that exaggerate the surface tension forces. As was pointed out in Chapter 6, edematous alveoli have a reduced volume. It is also possible that interstitial edema contributes to the abnormal stiffness of the lungs.

As would be expected from the histologic appearance of the lung (Figure 8.2), there is marked ventilation–perfusion inequality, with a substan-

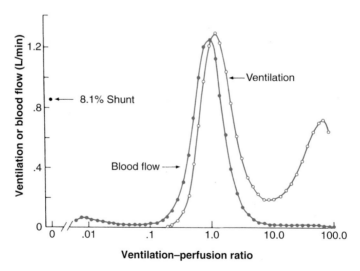

Figure 8.4. Distribution of ventilation–perfusion ratios in a patient who developed ARDS after a motor vehicle collision. Note the 8% shunt and the blood flow to units with low ventilation–perfusion ratios. In addition, there is some ventilation to high $\dot{V}_A/\dot{Q}$ units, probably as a result of the high airway pressure developed by the ventilator (compare Figure 10.3).

tial fraction of the total blood flow going to unventilated alveoli. This fraction may reach 50% or more. **Figure 8.4** shows some results obtained by the multiple inert gas method in a 44-year-old patient who developed respiratory failure after an automobile collision and who was mechanically ventilated. Note the presence of blood flow to lung units with abnormally low ventilation–perfusion ratios and also the shunt of 8% (compare the normal distribution in Figure 2.9). Figure 8.4 also shows a large amount of ventilation going to units with high ventilation–perfusion ratios. One reason for this is the abnormally high airway pressures developed by the ventilator, which reduce the blood flow in some alveoli (compare Figure 10.3).

The ventilation–perfusion inequality and shunt cause profound hypoxemia. In patients who have severe hypoxemia in spite of high concentrations of inspired oxygen, the Pa_{O_2}/FIO_2 is sometimes reported. Most patients require invasive mechanical ventilation during which they receive inspired oxygen concentrations between 40 and 100%. High levels of positive end-expiratory pressure (PEEP) are often necessary, and in very severe cases, other interventions including inhaled pulmonary vasodilators, ventilation in the prone position, neuromuscular blockade, and extracorporeal membrane oxygenation (ECMO) may be used to maintain an adequate arterial P_{O_2}.

The arterial P_{CO_2} varies significantly between patients. Some patients have a low or normal P_{CO_2} despite the severe ventilation–perfusion inequality and shunt, while others develop hypercarbia due to a significant increase in the physiologic dead space.

Infant Respiratory Distress Syndrome

This condition, which is also called hyaline membrane disease of the newborn, has several features in common with ARDS. Pathologically, the lung shows hemorrhagic edema, patchy atelectasis, and hyaline membranes caused by proteinaceous fluid and cellular debris within the alveoli. Physiologically, there is profound hypoxemia, with both ventilation–perfusion inequality and blood flow through unventilated lung. In addition, a right-to-left shunt via the patent foramen ovale may exaggerate the hypoxemia.

The chief cause of this condition is an absence of pulmonary surfactant, although other factors are also probably involved. The surfactant is normally produced by the type 2 alveolar epithelial cells (see Figure 5.2), and the ability of the lung to synthesize adequate amounts of the material develops relatively late in fetal life. Thus, a prematurely born infant is particularly at risk. The ability of the infant to secrete surfactant can be estimated by measuring the lecithin/sphingomyelin ratio of amniotic fluid, and maturation of the surfactant-synthesizing system can be hastened by the administration of corticosteroids to premature infants.

Treatment includes administration of exogenous surfactant as well as either nasal continuous positive airway pressure or invasive mechanical ventilation depending on the severity of the problem. High inspired oxygen concentrations and PEEP are often employed as well.

MANAGEMENT OF RESPIRATORY FAILURE

Although many factors might contribute to the respiratory failure of an individual patient, it is useful to discuss the physiologic principles that underlie a treatment. In addition to treating the underlying cause by, for example, giving antibiotics to a patient with pneumonia, there are several general factors that warrant attention when managing respiratory failure.

Hypoxemia

Hypoxemia is addressed by administering supplemental oxygen through one of a variety of different means described in detail in Chapter 9. The appropriate method varies based on the severity of the patient's illness.

Hypercapnia

While patients with hypoventilation due to a narcotic overdose can be treated with reversal agents like naloxone, most patients with hypercapnia require mechanical ventilatory support. This can be delivered either noninvasively through a tight-fitting mask or invasively through an endotracheal tube. These interventions are discussed in detail in Chapter 10.

Airway Resistance

Respiratory failure is often precipitated by an increase in airway resistance. Many patients have COPD of many years' duration with hypoxemia and even some mild hypercapnia. Even so, they are able to maintain some physical activity. However, if they develop bronchospasm through exposure to smog or cold air or if they have a respiratory infection with an increase in secretions and airway resistance, they may rapidly develop respiratory failure. The additional work of breathing becomes the straw that breaks the camel's back, and they develop profound hypoxemia, CO_2 retention, and respiratory acidosis.

Treatment should be directed at reducing the airway obstruction. Retained secretions are best removed by coughing when this is effective. Encouragement to cough and assistance by a respiratory therapist, nurse, or physician are often helpful, and changing the patient's position from side to side to assist drainage of secretions may be beneficial. Adequate hydration is important to prevent the secretions from becoming too viscid. Oxygen given by mechanical ventilation or facemask is often humidified to prevent thickening and crusting of secretions. Drugs such as aerosolized N-acetylcysteine to liquefy sputum are of doubtful value. Chest physiotherapy may help to clear airway secretions, while patients with neuromuscular weakness may benefit from use of mechanical insufflation–exsufflation devices. Any reversible airway obstruction should be treated by bronchodilators, such as albuterol or ipratropium, or perhaps intravenous corticosteroids. Care is necessary in the use of opiate medications. While they are effective at relieving dyspnea, they can also suppress cough and impair secretion clearance.

Compliance

The work of breathing may be increased due to reduced compliance from problems involving the lung parenchyma, chest wall, pleural space, and abdomen. In some cases, such as ARDS, compliance may only improve as the disease itself improves. In other cases, such as a patient with pulmonary edema and/or large pleural effusions, interventions such as diuresis or thoracentesis can lead to more rapid improvements in compliance and subsequent decreases in the work of breathing.

Respiratory Infection

Respiratory infections are a common precipitant of respiratory failure in patients with chronic lung disease. There are at least two physiologic mechanisms for this. First, the increased secretions and, perhaps, bronchospasm increase the work of breathing, as discussed earlier. Second, there is a worsening of ventilation–perfusion relationships so that even if the ventilation to the alveoli remains unchanged, there will be increasing hypoxemia and hypercapnia. For this reason, even when infection is not initially apparent, a careful search for sources of infection and prompt treatment with appropriate antimicrobial agents is indicated.

Cardiac Insufficiency

Many patients with severe chronic lung disease also have a compromised cardiovascular system. The pulmonary artery pressure is frequently raised as a result of several factors, including destruction of the pulmonary capillary bed by disease, hypoxic vasoconstriction, and perhaps increased blood viscosity caused by polycythemia. In addition, the myocardium is chronically hypoxic. Fluid retention often occurs as a result of retention of bicarbonate and sodium ions by the hypoxic kidney. Finally, some patients have coexisting coronary artery disease or cardiomyopathy. Identification and treatment of cardiac issues contributing to the patient's condition can speed resolution of their respiratory failure. For example, a patient with right heart failure due to severe COPD may benefit from treatment with diuretics.

KEY CONCEPTS

1. Respiratory failure refers to the condition when the lung fails to oxygenate the blood adequately or fails to prevent CO_2 retention.

2. The four causes of hypoxemia are hyperventilation, diffusion impairment, shunt, and ventilation–perfusion inequality, and the causes of CO_2 retention are hypoventilation and ventilation–perfusion inequality.

3. Severe hypoxemia causes many abnormalities including mental confusion, tachycardia, lactic acidosis, and proteinuria. CO_2 retention increases cerebral blood flow and may result in headache, confusion, or a decreased level of consciousness.

4. Gas exchange abnormalities in respiratory failure vary depending on the causative disease. For example, ARDS is characterized by severe hypoxemia with or without CO_2 retention. However, in pure hypoventilation, as in neuromuscular disease, CO_2 retention and respiratory acidosis dominate.

5. Management of respiratory failure involves treating the underlying cause, supporting oxygenation and ventilation, decreasing airway resistance, improving compliance, and treating infection and other contributing factors.

CLINICAL VIGNETTE

A 38-year-old woman with a history of chronic heavy alcohol use is admitted to the ICU with necrotizing pancreatitis. At the time of admission, she has an oxygen saturation of 97% breathing ambient air, a blood pressure of 89/67, and her chest radiograph shows no focal opacities. Following admission, she receives several liters of fluid to maintain an adequate mean arterial pressure. Four hours later, she complains of dyspnea, and her oxygen saturation is noted to be only 90% while breathing air. Despite starting her on oxygen by nasal cannula, her oxygen saturation continues to decrease, and she develops increased dyspnea. Due to her worsening clinical condition, she is intubated and started on invasive mechanical ventilation. A chest radiograph performed following intubation shows diffuse bilateral opacities (Figure 8.3). An echocardiogram shows normal left ventricular function. An arterial blood gas is performed while she is receiving 100% oxygen and shows a pH 7.45, Pa_{CO_2} 35, Pa_{O_2} 66, and HCO_3^- 22.

Questions
- Compared to the time of admission, what changes would you expect to see in her respiratory system compliance?
- What changes would you expect to see in her functional residual capacity?
- What is the most likely cause of her hypoxemia?
- Why is her Pa_{CO_2} low despite the severity of her respiratory failure?

QUESTIONS

1. A patient was admitted to the hospital with an exacerbation of chronic obstructive pulmonary disease. When given 100% oxygen to breathe, his arterial P_{CO_2} increased from 50 to 80 mm Hg. A likely cause was:

A. Increased airway resistance.
B. Depression of ventilation.
C. Depression of cardiac output.
D. Reduced levels of 2,3-diphosphoglycerate in the blood.
E. Bohr effect.

2. A 58-year-old woman with severe COPD due to long-standing smoking presents to the emergency department with worsening dyspnea and headache during a chest infection. On exam, she is confused and restless and has a flapping tremor and diffuse expiratory wheezes. Which of the following would you most likely see on an arterial blood gas in this patient?

A. Low pH with a primary respiratory acidosis
B. Low pH with a primary metabolic acidosis
C. High pH with a primary respiratory alkalosis
D. High pH with a primary metabolic alkalosis
E. Normal acid–base status

3. Following admission for injuries suffered in a motorcycle collision, a 41-year-old man develops worsening hypoxemia and requires mechanical ventilation with a high inspired oxygen fraction. A chest radiograph performed at the time of intubation reveals diffuse bilateral opacities. Which of the following changes in pulmonary function would you expect to see in this patient?

A. Increased lung compliance
B. Increased FRC
C. Increased shunt
D. Severe hypercarbia
E. Decreased airway resistance

4. Shortly after being born at only 31 week's gestation, a baby girl is noted to have nasal flaring, intercostal retractions, and hypoxemia on pulse oximetry. After a chest radiograph shows bilateral alveolar opacities, she is started on nasal continuous positive airway pressure. Which of the following medications should be also administered to speed resolution of her respiratory failure?

A. Digoxin
B. Diuretics
C. Inhaled albuterol
D. Inhaled ipratropium
E. Inhaled surfactant

5. A 71-year-old man with very severe COPD (FEV_1 ~28% predicted) presents with increasing cough, dyspnea, and sputum production following a viral upper respiratory infection. On examination, his S_pO_2 is 81% breathing air, and he has a prolonged expiratory phase and diffuse musical sounds on expiration. Which of the following physiologic changes are you most likely to see in his current clinical situation?
   A. Decreased airway resistance
   B. Increased ventilation–perfusion mismatch
   C. Increased arterial pH
   D. Reduced alveolar–arterial P_{O_2} difference
   E. Decreased arterial P_{CO_2}

OXYGEN THERAPY

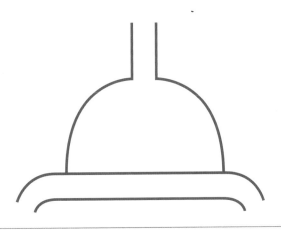

- **Improved Oxygenation After Oxygen Administration**
  Power of Added Oxygen
  Response of Various Types of
      Hypoxemia
      Hypoventilation
      Diffusion Impairment
      Ventilation–Perfusion
          Inequality
      Shunt
  Other Factors in Oxygen Delivery

- **Methods of Oxygen Administration**
  Nasal Cannulas
  Masks
  High-Flow Delivery Systems
  Transtracheal Oxygen
  Tents
  Ventilators
  Hyperbaric Oxygen
  Domiciliary and Portable Oxygen

- **Hazards of Oxygen Therapy**
  Carbon Dioxide Retention
  Oxygen Toxicity
  Atelectasis
      Following Airway Occlusion
      Instability of Units with Low
          Ventilation–Perfusion
          Ratios
  Retinopathy of Prematurity

Oxygen administration has a critical role in the treatment of hypoxemia and especially in the management of respiratory failure. However, patients vary considerably in their response to oxygen, and several potential hazards are associated with its use. A clear understanding of the physiologic principles involved is necessary to maximize its utility and minimize complications.

IMPROVED OXYGENATION AFTER OXYGEN ADMINISTRATION

Power of Added Oxygen

The great extent to which the arterial P_{O_2} can be increased by the inhalation of 100% oxygen is sometimes not appreciated. Suppose a young man has taken an overdose of a narcotic drug that results in severe hypoventilation with an arterial P_{O_2} of 50 mm Hg and a P_{CO_2} of 80 mm Hg (see Figure 2.2). If this patient is mechanically ventilated and given 100% oxygen, the arterial P_{O_2} may increase to over 600 mm Hg, that is, a 10-fold increase **(Figure 9.1)**. Few drugs can improve the gas composition of the blood so greatly and so effortlessly!

Response of Various Types of Hypoxemia

The mechanism of hypoxemia has an important bearing on its response to inhaled oxygen.

Hypoventilation

The rise in alveolar P_{O_2} can be predicted from the alveolar gas equation *if* the ventilation and metabolic rate, and therefore the alveolar P_{CO_2}, remain unaltered:

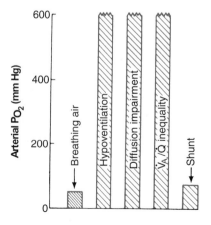

Figure 9.1. Response of the arterial P_{O_2} to 100% inspired oxygen for mechanisms of hypoxemia. The P_{O_2} breathing air is assumed to be 50 mm Hg. Note the dramatic increase in all instances except shunt where, nevertheless, there is a useful gain.

$$P_{A_{O_2}} = P_{I_{O_2}} - \frac{P_{A_{CO_2}}}{R} + F, \qquad \text{(Eq. 9.1)}$$

where F is a small correction factor.

Assuming no change in the alveolar P_{CO_2} and the respiratory exchange ratio, and neglecting the correction factor, this equation shows that the alveolar P_{O_2} rises in parallel with the inspired value. Thus, changing from air to only 30% oxygen can increase the alveolar P_{O_2} by approximately 60 mm Hg. In practice, the arterial P_{O_2} is always lower than the alveolar value because of a small amount of venous admixture. However, the hypoxemia of hypoventilation, which is rarely severe (see Figure 2.2), is easily reversed by a modest oxygen enrichment of the inspired gas. While oxygen is very effective in these cases, addressing the cause of hypoventilation is also important.

Diffusion Impairment
Again, hypoxemia caused by this mechanism is readily overcome by oxygen administration. The reason for this becomes clear if we look at the dynamics of oxygen uptake along the pulmonary capillary (see Figure 2.4). The rate of movement of oxygen across the blood–gas barrier is proportional to the P_{O_2} difference between alveolar gas and capillary blood. (See *West's Respiratory Physiology: The Essentials*. 10th ed. p. 29.) This difference is normally approximately 60 mm Hg at the beginning of the capillary. If we increase the concentration of inspired oxygen to only 30%, we raise the alveolar P_{O_2} by 60 mm Hg, thus doubling the rate of transfer of oxygen at the start of the capillary. This in turn improves oxygenation of the end-capillary blood. Therefore, a modest rise in inspired oxygen concentration can usually correct the hypoxemia.

Ventilation–Perfusion Inequality
Oxygen administration usually is very effective at improving the arterial P_{O_2} in this situation too. However, the rise in P_{O_2} depends on the pattern of ventilation–perfusion inequality and the inspired oxygen concentration. Administration of 100% O_2 increases the arterial P_{O_2} to high values because every lung unit that is ventilated eventually washes out its nitrogen. When this occurs, the alveolar P_{O_2} is given by $P_{O_2} = P_B - P_{H_2O} - P_{CO_2}$. Because the P_{CO_2} is normally less than 50 mm Hg, this equation predicts an alveolar P_{O_2} of over 600 mm Hg, even in lung units with very low ventilation–perfusion ratios.

However, two cautions should be added. First, some regions of the lung may be so poorly ventilated that it may take several minutes for the nitrogen to be washed out. Furthermore, these regions may continue to receive nitrogen as this gas is gradually washed out of peripheral tissues by the venous blood. As a consequence, the arterial P_{O_2} may take so long to reach its final level that, in practice, this is never achieved. Second, giving oxygen may result in the development of unventilated areas (Figure 9.5). If this occurs, the rise in arterial P_{O_2} stops short (Figure 9.3).

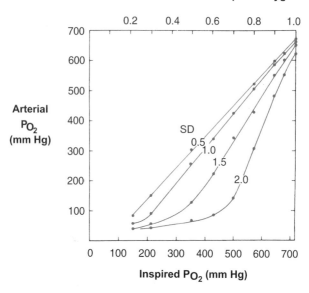

Figure 9.2. Response of the arterial P$_{O_2}$ to various inspired oxygen values in theoretical distributions of ventilation–perfusion ratios. *SD* refers to the standard deviation of the lognormal distribution. Note that when the distribution is broad (SD = 2), the arterial P$_{O_2}$ remains low even when 60% oxygen is inhaled. (From West JB, Wagner PD. Pulmonary gas exchange. In: West JB, ed. *Bioengineering Aspects of the Lung.* New York, NY: Marcel Dekker, 1977.)

When intermediate concentrations of oxygen are given, the rise in arterial P$_{O_2}$ is determined by the pattern of ventilation–perfusion inequality and in particular by those units that have low ventilation–perfusion ratios and appreciable blood flow. **Figure 9.2** shows the response of the arterial P$_{O_2}$ in lung models with various distributions of ventilation–perfusion ratios after inspiration of various oxygen concentrations. Note that at an inspired concentration of 60%, the arterial P$_{O_2}$ of the distribution with a standard deviation of 2.0 rose from 40 to only 90 mm Hg. This modest rise can be attributed to the effects of lung units with ventilation–perfusion ratios less than 0.01. For example, an alveolus with a ventilation–perfusion ratio of 0.006 that is given 60% O$_2$ to inspire has an end-capillary P$_{O_2}$ of only 60 mm Hg in the example shown. However, note that when the inspired oxygen concentration was increased to 90%, the arterial P$_{O_2}$ of this distribution rose to nearly 500 mm Hg.

Figure 9.2 assumes that the pattern of ventilation–perfusion inequality remains constant as the inspired oxygen is raised. However, the relief of alveolar hypoxia in poorly ventilated regions of the lung may increase the blood flow there because of the abolition of hypoxic vasoconstriction. In this case, the increase in arterial P$_{O_2}$ will be less. Note also that if units with low ventilation–perfusion ratios collapse during high oxygen breathing (Figure 9.5), the arterial P$_{O_2}$ rises less.

Shunt

This is the only mechanism of hypoxemia in which the arterial P_{O_2} remains far below the level for the normal lung during 100% O_2 breathing. The reason is that the blood that bypasses the ventilated alveoli (shunt) does not "see" the added oxygen and, being low in oxygen concentration, depresses the arterial P_{O_2}. This depression is particularly marked because of the nearly flat slope of the oxygen dissociation curve at a high P_{O_2} (see Figure 2.6).

However, it should be emphasized that useful gains in arterial P_{O_2} often follow the administration of 100% O_2 to patients with shunts. This is because of the additional dissolved oxygen, which can be appreciable at a high alveolar P_{O_2}. For example, increasing the alveolar P_{O_2} from 100 to 600 mm Hg raises the dissolved oxygen in the end-capillary blood from 0.3 to 1.8 mL of O_2/100 mL of blood. This increase of 1.5 mL of O_2/100 mL blood can be compared with the normal arterial–venous difference in oxygen concentration of approximately 5 mL/100 mL.

Figure 9.3 shows typical increases in arterial P_{O_2} for various percentage shunts at different inspired oxygen concentrations. The graph is drawn for an oxygen uptake of 300 mL/min and a cardiac output of 6 L/min; variations in these and other values alter the positions of the lines. However, in this example, a patient with a 30% shunt who has an arterial P_{O_2} of 55 mm Hg during air breathing increases this to 110 mm Hg if he or she breathes 100% oxygen. This increase corresponds to a rise in oxygen saturation and concentration of the arterial blood of 10% and 2.2 mL/100 mL, respectively. In a patient with a hypoxic myocardium, for example, these values mean an important gain in oxygen delivery.

Other Factors in Oxygen Delivery

Although the arterial P_{O_2} is a convenient measurement of the degree of oxygenation of the blood, other factors are important in oxygen delivery to the

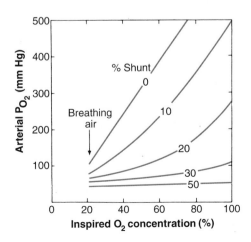

Figure 9.3. **Response of the arterial P_{O_2} to increased inspired oxygen concentrations in a lung with various amounts of shunt.** Note that the P_{O_2} remains far below the normal level for 100% oxygen. Nevertheless, useful gains in oxygenation occur even with severe degrees of shunting. (This diagram shows typical values only; changes in cardiac output, oxygen uptake, etc., affect the position of the lines.)

tissues. These factors include the hemoglobin concentration, the position of the oxygen dissociation curve, the cardiac output, and the distribution of the blood flow throughout the peripheral tissues.

Both a fall in hemoglobin concentration and cardiac output reduce the amount of oxygen per unit time ("oxygen flux") going to the tissues. The flux may be expressed as the product of the cardiac output and the arterial oxygen concentration: $\dot{Q} \times Ca_{O_2}$.

Diffusion of oxygen from the peripheral capillaries to the mitochondria in the tissue cells depends on capillary P_{O_2}. A useful index is the P_{O_2} of mixed venous blood, which reflects the average tissue P_{O_2}. A rearrangement of the Fick equation is as follows:

$$C\bar{v}_{O_2} = Ca_{O_2} - \frac{\dot{V}_{O_2}}{\dot{Q}} \qquad \text{(Eq. 9.2)}$$

This equation shows that the oxygen concentration (and therefore the P_{O_2}) of mixed venous blood will fall if either the arterial oxygen concentration or the cardiac output is reduced (oxygen consumption is assumed constant).

The relationship between oxygen concentration and P_{O_2} in the mixed venous blood depends on the position of the oxygen dissociation curve (see Figure 2.1). If the curve is shifted to the right by an increase in temperature, as in fever, or an increase in 2,3-diphosphoglycerate (DPG) concentration, as may occur in chronic hypoxemia, the P_{O_2} for a given concentration is high, thus favoring diffusion of oxygen to the mitochondria. By contrast, if the P_{CO_2} is low and the pH is high, as in respiratory alkalosis, or if the 2,3-DPG concentration is low because of transfusion of large amounts of stored blood, the resulting left-shifted curve interferes with oxygen unloading to the tissues.

Finally, the distribution of cardiac output clearly plays an important role in tissue oxygenation. For example, a patient who has coronary artery disease is liable to have hypoxic regions in the myocardium, irrespective of the other factors involved in oxygen delivery.

Important Factors in Oxygen Delivery to Tissues

- Arterial P_{O_2}
- Hemoglobin concentration
- Cardiac output
- Diffusion from capillaries to mitochondria (e.g., number of open capillaries)
- Oxygen affinity of hemoglobin
- Local blood flow

METHODS OF OXYGEN ADMINISTRATION

Nasal Cannulas

Nasal cannulas consist of two prongs that are inserted just inside the anterior nares and supported on a light frame. Oxygen is supplied at rates of 1 to 6 L/min, resulting in inspired oxygen concentrations of approximately 25% to 35%. The higher the patient's inspiratory flow rate, the lower the resulting concentration. When higher flow rates are used, the gas is often humidified to prevent patient discomfort and crusting of secretions on the nasal mucosa.

The chief advantage of cannulas is that the patient does not have the discomfort of a mask and he or she can talk and eat and has access to the face. The cannulas can be worn continuously for long periods, an important point because many patients with severe lung disease use oxygen on a chronic basis. The disadvantages of cannulas are the low maximum inspired concentrations of oxygen that are available and the unpredictability of the concentration, especially if the patient breathes with a high inspiratory flow rate or mostly through the mouth. This unpredictability can be minimized using a high-flow oxygen delivery system (see below).

Masks

Masks come in several designs. Simple plastic masks that fit over the nose and mouth allow inspired oxygen concentrations of up to 60% when supplied with flow rates of 10 to 15 L/min. Some patients report feeling smothered when this type of mask is used. Large holes in the side of the mask allow CO_2 to escape so it does not contribute to CO_2 retention.

Venturi masks are designed to deliver specific oxygen concentrations based on the Venturi effect. As oxygen enters the mask through a narrow jet, it entrains a constant flow of air, which enters via surrounding holes whose diameter can be adjusted to achieve the desired oxygen concentration. The smaller the diameter of the holes, the less ambient air in the gas mixture and the higher the inspired oxygen concentration. Masks that theoretically deliver inspired oxygen concentrations between 24% and 50% are available, but the true inspired concentration varies significantly between patients due to air leaks around the mask and variations in inspiratory flow rates.

Nonrebreather masks are designed to deliver high inspired oxygen concentrations approaching 80% to 100%. Oxygen is delivered at a flow rate of 10 to 15 L/min to a reservoir bag that hangs below the mask. Upon inhalation the patient draws oxygen-enriched air from this reservoir into their respiratory tract. Exhaled air escapes via one-way valves in the side of the mask designed to prevention inhalation of ambient air and reinhalation of exhaled air. As with the simple and venturi masks, air leaks and variations in inspiratory flow rate affect the delivered inspired oxygen concentration.

High-Flow Delivery Systems

Systems are now available for inhospital use that deliver oxygen at very high flow rates through either a facemask or nasal cannula. By delivering gas at flow rates as high as 60 L/min, the systems limit the entrainment of ambient air that leads to unpredictability of inspired oxygen concentrations in the systems described above. High-flow nasal cannula systems are also thought to have the added benefit of improving ventilatory efficiency by flushing of the dead space in the upper airway and generating some positive end-expiratory pressure (PEEP). In well-selected patients with acute hypoxemic respiratory failure, use of these systems may obviate the need for invasive mechanical ventilation.

Transtracheal Oxygen

Oxygen can be delivered via a microcatheter inserted through the anterior tracheal wall with the tip lying just above the carina. Although it is an efficient way of delivering oxygen, particularly for patients on long-term oxygen therapy, its clinical use has fallen off significantly due improvements in ambulatory oxygen systems used in the care of patients with chronic lung disease.

Tents

These are now used for children who do not tolerate masks well. Oxygen concentrations of up to 50% can be obtained, but there is a fire hazard.

Ventilators

When a patient is mechanically ventilated through an endotracheal or tracheostomy tube, complete control over the composition of the inspired gas is available. There is a theoretical risk of producing oxygen toxicity if concentrations of over 50% are given for more than 2 days (see later). In general, the lowest inspired oxygen that provides an acceptable arterial P_{O_2} should be used. This level is difficult to define, but in patients with acute respiratory distress syndrome (ARDS) who are being mechanically ventilated with high oxygen concentrations, a figure of 60 mm Hg is the typical goal.

Hyperbaric Oxygen

If 100% O_2 is administered at a pressure of three atmospheres, the inspired P_{O_2} is over 2,000 mm Hg. Under these conditions, a substantial increase in the arterial oxygen concentration can occur, chiefly as a result of additional dissolved oxygen. For example, if the arterial P_{O_2} is 2,000 mm Hg, the oxygen in solution is approximately 6 mL/100 mL of blood. Theoretically, this is enough to provide the entire arterial–venous difference of 5 mL/100 mL, so that the hemoglobin of the mixed venous blood could remain fully saturated.

Hyperbaric oxygen therapy has limited uses and is rarely indicated in the treatment of respiratory failure. However, it has been used in the treatment of severe carbon monoxide poisoning where most of the hemoglobin is unavailable to carry oxygen and therefore the dissolved oxygen is critically important. In addition, the high P_{O_2} accelerates the dissociation of carbon monoxide from hemoglobin. Severe anemic crises in patients who refuse blood transfusions are sometimes treated in the same way. Hyperbaric oxygen is sometimes used in the treatment of gas gangrene, nonhealing skin ulcers and as an adjunct to radiotherapy where the higher tissue P_{O_2} increases the radiosensitivity of relatively avascular tumors. The high-pressure chamber is also valuable for managing decompression sickness.

The use of hyperbaric oxygen requires a special facility with trained personnel. In practice, the chamber is filled with air, and oxygen is given by a special mask to ensure that the patient receives pure oxygen. This procedure also reduces fire hazard. Care is taken to avoid excessively high arterial P_{O_2}, which can provoke seizures.

Domiciliary and Portable Oxygen

Some patients are so disabled by severe chronic pulmonary disease that they are virtually confined to bed or a chair unless they breathe supplementary oxygen. These patients often benefit considerably from having a supply of oxygen in their home. Oxygen can be delivered using a large tank or an oxygen concentrator, which extracts oxygen from the air using a synthetic zeolite that preferentially absorbs nitrogen. Most patients also use portable oxygen sets to facilitate travel outside the home that use either liquid oxygen as a store or an oxygen concentrator.

The patients who benefit most from portable oxygen are those whose exercise tolerance is limited by dyspnea. Increasing the inspired oxygen concentration can greatly increase the level of exercise for a given ventilation and so enable these patients to become much more active.

It has been shown that a low flow of oxygen given continuously can reduce the amount of pulmonary hypertension and improve the prognosis of some patients with advanced chronic obstructive pulmonary disease (COPD). Although such therapy is expensive, improvements in the technology of providing oxygen have made it increasingly feasible for many patients.

HAZARDS OF OXYGEN THERAPY

Carbon Dioxide Retention

The reasons for the development of dangerous CO_2 retention after oxygen administration to patients with severe COPD or the obesity hypoventilation syndrome were briefly discussed in Chapter 8. A critical factor in the ventilatory drive of these patients who have a high work of breathing is often the hypoxic stimulation of their peripheral chemoreceptors. If this is removed by relieving their hypoxemia, the level of ventilation may fall precipitously and severe CO_2 retention may ensue. Relief of hypoxic pulmonary vasoconstriction and changes in ventilation–perfusion matching also play an important role.

In patients with CO_2 retention, intermittent use or abrupt cessation of supplemental oxygen can lead to dangerous severe hypoxemia. The physiologist Haldane compared intermittent use, for example, with bringing a drowning man to the surface—occasionally! The explanation is that if oxygen administration is seen to cause CO_2 retention and is abruptly stopped, the subsequent hypoxemia may be more severe than it was before oxygen therapy. The reason is the increased alveolar P_{CO_2}, as can be seen from the alveolar gas equation:

$$P_{A_{O_2}} = P_{I_{O_2}} - \frac{P_{A_{CO_2}}}{R} + F \qquad \text{(Eq. 9.3)}$$

This shows that any increase in alveolar P_{CO_2} will reduce the alveolar P_{O_2} and therefore the arterial value. Moreover, the high P_{CO_2} is likely to remain for many minutes because the body stores of this gas are so great that the excess is washed out only gradually. Thus, the hypoxemia may be severe and prolonged.

These patients should be given continuous oxygen at a low concentration to achieve an oxygen saturation of 88% to 94%, with monitoring of ventilation using end-tidal CO_2 monitoring or arterial blood gases. The shape of the oxygen dissociation curve (see Figure 2.1) should be at the back of the physician's mind to remind him or her that a rise in P_{O_2} from 30 to 50 mm Hg (at a normal pH) represents more than a 25% increase in hemoglobin saturation!

Oxygen Toxicity

Animal studies have demonstrated that high concentrations of oxygen over long periods damage the lung. Studies of monkeys exposed to 100% oxygen for 2 days show that some of the earliest changes are in the capillary endothelial cells, which become swollen. Alterations occur in the endothelial intercellular junctions, and there is an increased capillary permeability that leads to interstitial and alveolar edema. In addition, the alveolar epithelium may become denuded and replaced by rows of type 2 epithelial cells. Later, organization occurs with interstitial fibrosis.

The extent to which these changes occur in humans is difficult to determine but normal subjects report substernal discomfort after breathing 100% oxygen for 24 hours. Patients who have been mechanically ventilated with 100% oxygen for 36 hours have shown a progressive fall in arterial P_{O_2} compared with a control group who were ventilated with air. In practice, such high levels over such a long period can be achieved only in patients who are intubated and mechanically ventilated. The risks of using high inspired oxygen concentrations must be balanced against the need to maintain adequate arterial oxygenation in patients with severe hypoxemic respiratory failure. For this reason, the general practice is to use the lowest inspired oxygen concentration necessary to maintain an adequate arterial P_{O_2}.

Atelectasis

Following Airway Occlusion

If a patient is breathing air and an airway becomes totally obstructed, for example, by retained secretions, absorption atelectasis of the lung behind the airway may occur. The reason is that the sum of the partial pressures in the venous blood is less than atmospheric pressure, with the result that the trapped gas is gradually absorbed. (See *West's Respiratory Physiology: The Essentials*. 10th ed. pp. 168–169.) However, the process is relatively slow, requiring many hours or even days.

However, if the patient is breathing a high concentration of oxygen, the rate of absorption atelectasis is greatly accelerated. This is because there is then relatively little nitrogen in the alveoli and this gas normally slows the absorption process because of its low solubility. Replacing the nitrogen with any other gas that is rapidly absorbed also predisposes to collapse. An example is nitrous oxide during anesthesia. In the normal lung, collateral ventilation may delay or prevent atelectasis by providing an alternative path for gas to enter the obstructed region (see Figure l.11C).

Absorption atelectasis is common in patients with respiratory failure because they often have excessive secretions or cellular debris in their airways and they are frequently treated with high oxygen concentrations. In addition, the channels through which collateral ventilation normally occurs may be obstructed by disease. Collapse is common in the dependent regions of the lung because secretions tend to collect there, and those airways and alveoli are relatively poorly expanded anyway (see Figure 3.4). Hypoxemia develops to the extent that atelectatic lung is perfused, although hypoxic vasoconstriction may limit this to some extent.

Instability of Units with Low Ventilation–Perfusion Ratios

It has been shown that lung units with low ventilation–perfusion ratios may become unstable and collapse when high oxygen mixtures are inhaled. An example is given in **Figure 9.4**, which shows the distribution of ventilation–perfusion ratios in a patient during air breathing and after 30 minutes of 100% oxygen. This patient had respiratory failure after an automobile collision (see Figure 8.4). Note that during air breathing, there were appreciable amounts of blood flow to lung units with low ventilation–perfusion ratios in addition to an 8% shunt. After oxygen administration, the blood flow to the low ventilation–perfusion ratio units was not evident, but the shunt had increased to nearly 16%. The most likely explanation of this change is that the poorly ventilated regions became unventilated.

Figure 9.5 shows the mechanism involved. The figure shows four hypothetical lung units, all with low inspired ventilation–perfusion ratios ($\dot{V}_A/\dot{Q}$) during 80% oxygen breathing. In A, the inspired (alveolar) ventilation is 49.4 units, but the expired ventilation is only 2.5 units (the actual values depend on the blood flow). The reason why so little gas is exhaled is that so

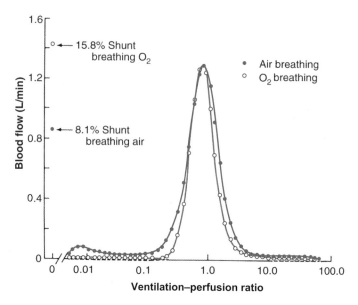

Figure 9.4. **Conversion of low ventilation–perfusion ratio units to shunt during oxygen breathing.** This patient had respiratory failure after an automobile collision (same patient as shown in Figure 8.3). During air breathing, there was appreciable blood flow to units with low ventilation–perfusion ratios. After 30 minutes of 100% oxygen, blood flow to these units was not evident, but the shunt doubled.

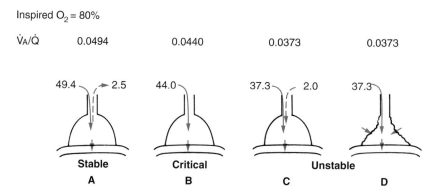

Figure 9.5. **Mechanism of the collapse of lung units with low inspired ventilation–perfusion ratios ($\dot{V}_A/\dot{Q}$) when high oxygen mixtures are inhaled. A.** The expired ventilation is very small because so much of the inspired gas is taken up by the blood. **B.** There is no expired ventilation because all of the ventilation is taken up by the blood. **C, D.** More gas is removed from the lung unit than is inspired, leading to an unstable condition.

much is taken up by the blood. In B, where the inspired ventilation is slightly reduced to 44.0 units (same blood flow as before), there is no expired ventilation because all the gas that is inspired is absorbed by the blood. Such a unit is said to have a "critical" ventilation–perfusion ratio.

In Figure 9.5C and D, the inspired ventilation has been further reduced with the result that it is now less than the volume of gas entering the blood. This is an unstable situation. Under these circumstances, either gas is inspired from neighboring units during the expiratory phase of respiration, as in C, or the unit gradually collapses, as in D. The latter fate is particularly likely if the unit is poorly ventilated because of intermittent airway closure. This is probably common in the dependent regions of the lung in ARDS because of the greatly reduced FRC. The likelihood of atelectasis increases rapidly as the inspired oxygen concentration approaches 100%.

The development of shunts during oxygen breathing is an additional reason to avoid, if possible, high concentrations of this gas in the treatment of patients with respiratory failure. Also, the shunt that is measured during 100% oxygen breathing (see Figure 2.6) in these patients may substantially overestimate the shunt that is present during air breathing.

Retinopathy of Prematurity

If premature infants with the infant respiratory distress syndrome are treated with high concentrations of oxygen, they may develop fibrosis behind the lens of the eye, leading to retinal detachment and blindness. Formerly known as retrolental fibroplasia, this problem can be prevented by avoiding overly high arterial P_{O_2} and other established risk factors.

KEY CONCEPTS

1. Oxygen therapy is extremely valuable in the treatment of many patients with lung disease, and it can often greatly increase the arterial P_{O_2}.

2. The response of the arterial P_{O_2} to inhaled oxygen varies considerably depending on the cause of the hypoxemia. Patients with large shunts do not respond well, although even here the increase in arterial P_{O_2} can be helpful.

3. Various methods of oxygen administration are available. Nasal cannulas are valuable for long-term treatment of patients with COPD. The highest inspired oxygen concentrations are obtained with intubation and mechanical ventilation.

4. Hazards of oxygen therapy include oxygen toxicity, carbon dioxide retention, atelectasis, and retinopathy of prematurity.

CLINICAL VIGNETTE

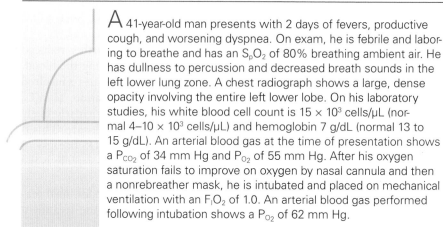

A 41-year-old man presents with 2 days of fevers, productive cough, and worsening dyspnea. On exam, he is febrile and laboring to breathe and has an S_pO_2 of 80% breathing ambient air. He has dullness to percussion and decreased breath sounds in the left lower lung zone. A chest radiograph shows a large, dense opacity involving the entire left lower lobe. On his laboratory studies, his white blood cell count is 15×10^3 cells/μL (normal $4–10 \times 10^3$ cells/μL) and hemoglobin 7 g/dL (normal 13 to 15 g/dL). An arterial blood gas at the time of presentation shows a P_{CO_2} of 34 mm Hg and P_{O_2} of 55 mm Hg. After his oxygen saturation fails to improve on oxygen by nasal cannula and then a nonrebreather mask, he is intubated and placed on mechanical ventilation with an F_IO_2 of 1.0. An arterial blood gas performed following intubation shows a P_{O_2} of 62 mm Hg.

Questions

- How do you explain the observed change in his P_{O_2} following initiation of mechanical ventilation?
- What effect will his fever have on tissue oxygen delivery?
- What change would you expect to see in his mixed venous oxygen content compared to his normal healthy state?
- What interventions besides mechanical ventilation with a high inspired oxygen concentration can be considered to improve tissue oxygen delivery?

QUESTIONS

1. A previously well young man was admitted to the emergency department with a benzodiazepine overdose that caused severe hypoventilation. When he was given 50% oxygen to breathe, there was no change in his arterial P_{CO_2}. Approximately how much would his arterial P_{O_2} (mm Hg) be expected to rise?
   A. 25
   B. 50
   C. 75
   D. 100
   E. 200

2. A patient with congenital heart disease has a right-to-left shunt of 20% of the cardiac output and an arterial P_{O_2} of 60 mm Hg during air breathing. When he is given 100% oxygen to breathe, you would expect his arterial P_{O_2} to:
   A. Fall.
   B. Remain unchanged.
   C. Increase by less than 10 mm Hg.
   D. Increase by more than 10 mm Hg.
   E. Rise to about 600 mm Hg.

3. A blood sample from a patient with carbon monoxide poisoning showed a reduction in P_{50} of the oxygen dissociation curve. The probable reason was:
   A. Increased arterial P_{O_2}.
   B. Carbon monoxide's effect on hemoglobin's oxygen affinity.
   C. Increased red blood cell 2,3-DPG concentration.
   D. Reduced arterial pH.
   E. Mild pyrexia.

4. A disadvantage of nasal cannulas for oxygen administration compared with masks is:
   A. They are more uncomfortable than masks.
   B. Inspired oxygen concentrations above 25% are impossible to obtain.
   C. The inspired oxygen concentration varies considerably.
   D. The patient cannot talk.
   E. The inspired P_{CO_2} tends to rise.

5. A patient with normal lungs but severe anemia is placed in a hyperbaric chamber, total pressure three atmospheres, and 100% oxygen is administered by valve box. You can expect the dissolved oxygen in the arterial blood (in mL O_2/100 mL blood) to increase to:
   A. 1.
   B. 2.
   C. 3.
   D. 4.
   E. 6.

6. Lung units with low ventilation–perfusion ratios may collapse when high concentrations of oxygen are inhaled for 1 hour, because:
   A. Pulmonary surfactant is inactivated.
   B. Oxygen toxicity causes alveolar edema.
   C. Gas is taken up by the blood faster than it can enter the units by ventilation.
   D. Interstitial edema around the small airways causes airway closure.
   E. Inflammatory changes occur in the small airways.

7. A 71-year-old man with very severe COPD is admitted to the hospital with an exacerbation of his disease. After he is placed on 6 L/min of oxygen by nasal cannula, his S_pO_2 increases from 80% breathing air to 99%. Two hours later, he is noted to be more somnolent and an arterial blood gas reveals that his Pa_{CO_2} rose from 48 mm Hg on admission to 59 mm Hg. Which of the following statements best explains the observed change in his Pa_{CO_2}?
   A. Decreased peripheral chemoreceptor stimulation of ventilation
   B. Improved ventilation–perfusion matching
   C. Rightward shift of the hemoglobin–oxygen dissociation curve
   D. Increased formation of carbamino groups on the hemoglobin chains
   E. Increased arterial pH

MECHANICAL VENTILATION

10

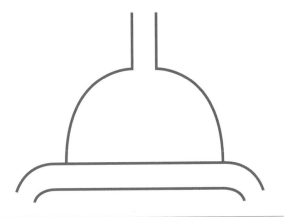

- **Methods of Mechanical Ventilation**
  Invasive Mechanical Ventilation
  Noninvasive Mechanical Ventilation
  Tank Ventilators

- **When to Initiate Mechanical Ventilation**

- **Modes of Mechanical Ventilation**
  Volume Control
  Pressure Control
  Pressure Support
  Continuous Positive Airway Pressure
  High-Frequency Ventilation

- **Positive End-Expiratory Pressure**

- **Physiologic Effects of Mechanical Ventilation**
  Reduction of Arterial P_{CO_2}
  Increase in Arterial P_{O_2}
  Effects on Venous Return
  Miscellaneous Hazards

Mechanical ventilation is of major importance in treating patients with respiratory failure. Once used only as an emergency procedure in resuscitation or as a last resort in the treatment of the critically ill, it is now frequently employed to support patients with respiratory failure. Mechanical ventilation is a complex and technical subject, and this discussion is limited to the physiologic principles of its use, benefits, and hazards.

METHODS OF MECHANICAL VENTILATION

Mechanical ventilation can be delivered to patients through a variety of means.

Invasive Mechanical Ventilation

The majority of patients with acute respiratory failure are supported through invasive mechanical ventilation in which the ventilator is connected to the upper airway via an endotracheal or, less commonly, a tracheostomy tube. The latter is usually placed after a patient has been endotracheally intubated for a long period of time but is occasionally placed at the onset of respiratory failure when the upper airway is compromised by, for example, anaphylaxis or a laryngeal tumor. These tubes include an inflatable cuff at the distal end to give an airtight seal. Endotracheal tubes can be inserted via the nose or mouth. With either type of tube, the lungs are inflated by delivering positive pressure to the airway **(Figure 10.1)**.

Noninvasive Mechanical Ventilation

Positive pressure can also be applied to the airway using a tight-fitting mask around the patient's nose and mouth. This noninvasive form of support is

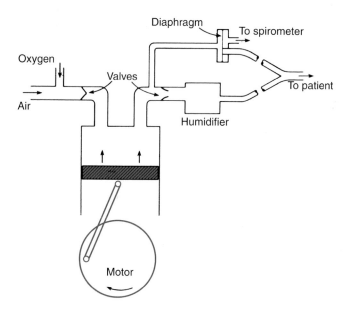

Figure 10.1. Example of a constant-volume ventilation (schematic). In practice, the tidal volume and frequency can be regulated. During the expiratory phase, as the piston descends, the diaphragm is deflected to the left by the reduced pressure in the cylinder, allowing the patient to exhale through the spirometer.

increasingly being used in critical care, particularly for patients with acute exacerbations of chronic obstructive pulmonary disease, the obesity hypoventilation syndrome, and other forms of ventilatory failure where the duration of need for ventilatory support is expected to be short. It is not an effective form of support, however, for patients with severe hypoxemic respiratory failure due to pneumonia or the acute respiratory distress syndrome (ARDS) and is generally avoided in patients who cannot protect their airway, who have excessive respiratory secretions or who are at high risk for aspiration.

Tank Ventilators

Unlike with the methods described above, tank respirators deliver negative pressure (less than atmospheric) to the outside of the chest and rest of the body, excluding the head. They consist of a rigid box (iron lung) connected to a large-volume, low-pressure pump that controls the respiratory cycle. The box is often hinged along the middle so that it can be opened to allow nursing care.

Tank ventilators are no longer used in the treatment of acute respiratory failure because they limit access to the patient and because they are bulky and inconvenient. They were employed extensively to ventilate patients with bulbar poliomyelitis, and they are still occasionally useful for patients with chronic neuromuscular disease who need to be ventilated for months or years. A modification of the tank ventilator is the cuirass, which fits over the thorax and abdomen and also generates negative pressure. It is usually reserved for patients who have partially recovered from neuromuscular respiratory failure.

WHEN TO INITIATE MECHANICAL VENTILATION

The decision to initiate mechanical ventilation should not be lightly undertaken because it is a major intervention that requires a substantial investment of personnel and equipment, with many hazards. There are no specific numerical thresholds for the arterial P_{CO_2} or P_{O_2} that mandate mechanical support. Instead, the timing of mechanical ventilation is dictated by factors such as the severity of the disease process, the rapidity of the progress of hypoxemia and hypercapnia, and the hemodynamic stability and general condition of the patient.

MODES OF MECHANICAL VENTILATION

The majority of modern ventilators can deliver positive-pressure ventilation by a variety of means, referred to as "modes" of ventilation. The appropriate mode for a given patient varies based on their clinical and physiologic needs.

Volume Control

A preset volume is delivered to the patient at a specified rate. However, patients who are not paralyzed and have normal respiratory muscles can initiate breaths beyond the set rate and receive the full tidal volume with each extra breath. The ratio of inspiratory to expiratory time can also be controlled. This can be particularly useful in patients with obstructive lung disease for whom it is important to ensure adequate time for exhalation.

This mode has the advantage of having a known volume delivered to the patient despite changes in the elastic properties of the lung or chest wall or increases in airway resistance. A disadvantage is that high pressures can be developed. However, in practice, a safety blow-off valve prevents pressures from reaching dangerous levels.

Pressure Control

Rather than delivering a constant tidal volume with each breath, this mode delivers a preset pressure for a specified duration of time. A minimum frequency is set, but patients can initiate breaths beyond the specified rate, during which they receive the preset pressure. The flow of gas is not set by the practitioner and, instead, is determined by the change in pressure on inhalation and airway resistance. The ratio of inspiratory to expiratory time is controlled by adjusting the inspiratory time.

The advantage of this mode is that it prevents development of excessive airway pressure. The chief disadvantage is that the volume of gas delivered with each breath can vary with changes in the compliance of the respiratory system. Also, an increase in airway resistance may decrease the ventilation because there may be insufficient time for equilibration of pressure between the machine and the alveoli. Minute ventilation must therefore be monitored closely by following the Pa_{CO_2} on arterial blood gases.

Pressure Support

This mode is similar to pressure control in that the patient receives the preset pressure during inhalation. However, there is no preset rate, and the patient must initiate all of the breaths. As such, it is only suitable for patients who are able to initiate breathing. In addition, rather than being turned off after a preset time, the inspiratory pressure is terminated once inspiratory flow falls below a certain threshold. This mode, which is commonly used for patients who require intubation solely to prevent aspiration of oral or gastric secretions or are having difficulty being liberated from the ventilator due to neuromuscular weakness, is generally more comfortable for patients.

A variant of this mode, referred to as bilevel positive airway pressure, is commonly used during noninvasive mechanical ventilation. When the patient initiates a breath, the inspiratory pressure is raised to and maintained at a preset level, referred to as the inspiratory positive airway pressure (IPAP) until inspiratory flow decreases. During exhalation, airway pressure is maintained at a level above zero cm H_2O, referred to as the expiratory positive airway pressure (EPAP), which serves the same function as positive end-expiratory pressure (PEEP, discussed below).

Continuous Positive Airway Pressure

In this mode, a constant positive pressure is applied to the airway by the ventilator during inhalation and exhalation. This improves oxygenation by increasing functional residual capacity (FRC) and preventing atelectasis. Continuous positive airway pressure (CPAP) is commonly used in patients being weaned from ventilator breathing or who are intubated solely for airway protection.

It can also be applied to patients through a tight-fitting mask, as is done in neonates with infant respiratory distress syndrome (see Chapter 8) or adults with acute heart failure exacerbations.

High-Frequency Ventilation

In high-frequency jet or oscillatory ventilation, very low tidal volumes (50 to 100 mL) are delivered at a high frequency (approximately 20 cycles per second). The lung is vibrated rather than expanded in the conventional way, and the transport of the gas occurs by a combination of diffusion and convection. Because it maintains higher mean airway pressures than more conventional ventilator modes, high-frequency ventilation is sometimes used in patients with severe ARDS, although this practice is more common in children than adults. Another use is in patients with gas leaks from the lung via a bronchopleural fistula.

POSITIVE END-EXPIRATORY PRESSURE

For most patients receiving mechanical ventilation, 5 cm H_2O of pressure is applied to the airways during exhalation. This is referred to as positive end-expiratory pressure (PEEP) and is designed to counteract the decrease in FRC and atelectasis that can occur when patients are ventilated in the supine or semirecumbent position. Rather than being a mode of mechanical ventilation per se, it is an intervention that can be used in most modes of mechanical ventilatory support.

When the arterial P_{O_2} does not rise despite increased inspired oxygen concentrations, as can happen in patients with large shunts due to severe pneumonia or ARDS (See Figure 9.3), PEEP is often raised to levels higher than 5 cm H_2O as a means to improve gas exchange. In some cases, pressures as high as 20 cm H_2O may be used. Several mechanisms are probably responsible for the increase in arterial P_{O_2} with increased PEEP. The positive pressure increases the transpulmonary pressure and, as a result, increases functional residual capacity (FRC), which is typically small in these patients because of the increased elastic recoil of the lung. By doing so, PEEP reverses the low lung volumes that lead to airway closure, intermittent or absent ventilation and absorption atelectasis, especially in the dependent regions (see Figures 3.4 and 9.5). Patients with edema in their airways also benefit, probably because the fluid is moved into small peripheral airways or alveoli, allowing some regions of the lung to be reventilated. A secondary gain from PEEP is that it may allow the inspired oxygen concentration to be decreased, thus lessening the risk of oxygen toxicity.

Positive End-Expiratory Pressure (PEEP)

- Increases FRC and prevents atelectasis.
- 5 cm H_2O used in most patients receiving mechanical ventilation.
- Higher levels useful for raising the arterial P_{O_2} in patients with respiratory failure.
- Values as high as 20 cm H_2O can be used in cases of severe hypoxemia.
- May allow the inspired O_2 concentration to be reduced.

PHYSIOLOGIC EFFECTS OF MECHANICAL VENTILATION

Reduction of Arterial P_{CO2}

A major role of mechanical ventilation is to decrease the P_{CO_2}, which may have been elevated because the patient is not able to breathe spontaneously, as in neuromuscular disease or a drug overdose, or because the lung itself is severely diseased, as in ARDS. In patients with airway obstruction in whom the oxygen cost of breathing is high, mechanical ventilation may appreciably reduce the oxygen uptake and CO_2 output, thus contributing to the fall in arterial P_{CO_2}.

The relationship between the arterial P_{CO_2} and the alveolar ventilation in normal lungs is given by the alveolar ventilation equation:

$$P_{CO_2} = \frac{\dot{V}_{CO_2}}{\dot{V}_A} \cdot K \qquad \text{(Eq. 10.1)}$$

where K is a constant. In diseased lungs, the denominator $\dot{V}_A$ in this equation is less than the ventilation going to the alveoli because of alveolar dead space, that is, unperfused alveoli or those with high ventilation–perfusion ratios. For this reason, the denominator is sometimes referred to as the "effective alveolar ventilation."

Mechanical ventilation frequently increases both the alveolar and anatomic dead spaces. As a consequence, the effective alveolar ventilation is not increased as much as the total ventilation. This is particularly likely if high pressures are applied to the airway. This can be seen in the example shown in

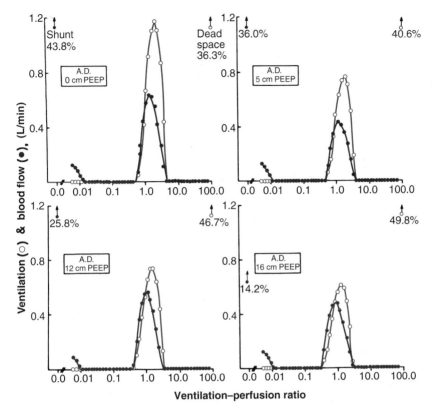

Figure 10.2. Reduction of shunt and increase of dead space caused by increasing levels of PEEP in a patient with acute respiratory distress syndrome (ARDS). Note that as the PEEP was progressively increased from 0 to 16 cm H$_2$O, the shunt decreased from 43.8 to 14.2% of the cardiac output, and the dead space increased from 36.3 to 49.8% of the tidal volume. (From Dantzker DR, Brook CJ, DeHart P, et al. Ventilation–perfusion distributions in the adult respiratory distress syndrome. *Am Rev Respir Dis* 1979;120:1039–1052.)

Figure 10.2. As the level of PEEP was increased from 0 to 16 cm H$_2$O in this patient with ARDS, the dead space increased from 36.3 to 49.8%. In some patients, high levels of PEEP also result in the appearance of lung units with high ventilation–perfusion ratios that cause a shoulder to form on the right of the ventilation distribution curve. This did not occur in the example shown. Occasionally, a large physiologic dead space is seen with positive-pressure ventilation even in the absence of PEEP. An example is shown in Figure 8.4.

There are several reasons why positive-pressure ventilation increases dead space. First, lung volume is usually raised, especially when PEEP is added, and the resulting radial traction on the airways increases the anatomic dead space. Next, the raised airway pressure tends to divert blood flow away from ventilated regions, thus causing areas of high ventilation–perfusion ratio or even unperfused areas **(Figure 10.3)**. This is particularly likely to happen in

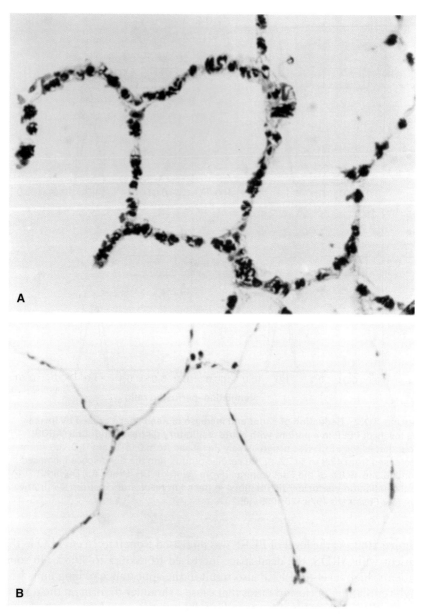

Figure 10.3. Effect of raised airway pressure on the histologic appearance of pulmonary capillaries. A. Normal appearance. **B.** Collapse of capillaries when alveolar pressure is raised above capillary pressure. (From Glazier JB, Hughes JMB, Maloney JE, et al. Measurements of capillary dimensions and blood volume in rapidly frozen lungs. *J Appl Physiol* 1969;26:65–76.)

the uppermost regions of the lung where the pulmonary artery pressure is relatively low because of the hydrostatic effect. (See *West's Respiratory Physiology: The Essentials*. 10th ed. p. 50). Indeed, if the pressure in the capillaries falls below airway pressure, the capillaries may collapse completely, resulting in unperfused lung (Figure 10.3). This collapse is encouraged by two factors: (1) the abnormally high airway pressure and (2) the reduced venous return and consequent hypoperfusion of the lung. The latter is particularly likely to occur if there is a reduced circulating blood volume (see later in this chapter).

The tendency for the arterial P_{CO_2} to rise as a result of the increased dead space can be countered by increasing the respiratory rate to increase the total ventilation. Nevertheless, it is important to remember that an increase in mean airway pressure can cause a substantial rise in dead space, although the increased pressure may be necessary to combat the shunt and resulting hypoxemia (Figure 10.2).

In practice, some patients who are mechanically ventilated develop an abnormally low arterial P_{CO_2} because they are overventilated. This results in a respiratory alkalosis that frequently coexists with a metabolic acidosis because of the hypoxemia and impaired peripheral circulation. An unduly low arterial P_{CO_2} should be avoided because it reduces cerebral blood flow and may cause cerebral hypoxia.

Another hazard of overventilation of patients with CO_2 retention is a low serum potassium, which predisposes to arrhythmia. When CO_2 is retained, potassium moves out of the cells into the plasma and is excreted by the kidney. If the P_{CO_2} is then rapidly reduced, the potassium moves back into the cells, thus depleting the plasma.

Increase in Arterial P_{O_2}

In many patients with respiratory failure, the primary objective of mechanical ventilation is to increase the arterial P_{O_2}. In practice, such patients are always ventilated with oxygen-enriched mixtures. The inspired oxygen concentration should ideally be sufficient to raise the arterial P_{O_2} to at least 60 mm Hg, but unduly high inspired concentrations should be avoided because of the hazards of oxygen toxicity and atelectasis. As noted above, increased inspired oxygen concentrations may not increase the Pa_{O_2} in patients with large shunts, and PEEP is necessary to improve the situation.

Figure 10.2 shows the effects of PEEP in a patient with ARDS. Note that the level of PEEP was progressively increased from 0 to 16 cm H_2O, and this caused the shunt to fall from 43.8% to 14.2% of the cardiac output. A small amount of blood flow to poorly ventilated alveoli remained. The increase in PEEP also caused the dead space to increase from 36.3% to 49.8% of the tidal volume. This can be explained by compression of the capillaries by the increased alveolar pressure and also the increase in volume of the lung and consequent increased radial traction on the airways, which increases their volume. This situation is discussed further below.

Occasionally, the addition of too much PEEP reduces rather than increases the arterial P_{O_2}. One important mechanism is a substantial fall in cardiac output on high levels of PEEP, which reduces the P_{O_2} of mixed venous blood and therefore the arterial P_{O_2}. PEEP tends to reduce cardiac output by impeding venous return to the thorax, especially if the circulating blood volume has been depleted by hemorrhage or shock. Accordingly, its value should not be gauged by its effect on the arterial P_{O_2} alone but in terms of the total amount of oxygen delivered to the tissues. The product of the arterial oxygen concentration and the cardiac output is a useful index because changes in this alter the P_{O_2} of mixed venous blood and therefore the P_{O_2} of many tissues.

Other mechanisms by which PEEP may reduce the P_{O_2} include reduced ventilation of well-perfused regions (because of increasing dead space and ventilation to poorly perfused regions) and diversion of blood flow away from ventilated to unventilated regions by the raised airway pressure. The latter problem is often observed when PEEP is used in processes with focal, rather than diffuse, lung involvement.

Another hazard of high levels of PEEP is damage to the pulmonary capillaries as a result of the high tension in the alveolar walls. The alveolar wall can be considered a string of capillaries. High levels of tension greatly increase the stresses on the capillary walls, causing disruption of the alveolar epithelium, capillary endothelium, or sometimes all layers of the wall. This is another example of "stress failure," which was discussed in Chapter 6 in relation to pulmonary edema caused by high capillary hydrostatic pressures.

Effects on Venous Return

As noted above, mechanical ventilation tends to impede the return of blood into the thorax and thus reduce the cardiac output. This is true for both positive-pressure and negative-pressure ventilation. In a supine, relaxed patient, the return of blood to the thorax depends on the difference between the peripheral venous pressure and the mean intrathoracic pressure. If the airway pressure is increased by a ventilator, mean intrathoracic pressure rises, and venous return is impeded. Even if airway pressure remains atmospheric, as in a tank respirator, venous return tends to fall because the peripheral venous pressure is reduced by the negative pressure. Only with the cuirass respirator is venous return virtually unaffected.

The effects of positive-pressure ventilation on venous return depend on the magnitude and duration of the inspiratory pressure, and particularly, on the addition of PEEP. The ideal pattern from this standpoint is a short inspiratory phase of relatively low pressure followed by a long expiratory phase and zero (or slightly negative) end-expiratory pressure. However, such a pattern encourages a low lung volume and consequent hypoxemia, and a compromise is generally necessary. The 5 cm H_2O of PEEP given to most patients receiving mechanical ventilation generally has little effect on venous return.

An important determinant of venous return is the magnitude of the circulating blood volume. If this is reduced, for example, by hemorrhage or shock, positive-pressure ventilation often causes a marked fall in cardiac output. Systemic hypotension may ensue. It is therefore important to correct any volume depletion by appropriate fluid replacement. The central venous pressure is often monitored as a guide to this but should be interpreted in the light of the increased airway pressure. Positive airway pressure itself raises central venous pressure.

Venous return may also decrease due to a process referred to as "auto-PEEP." If the patient is unable to completely exhale the delivered tidal volume with each breath, progressive hyperinflation can develop leading to an increase in intrathoracic pressure and decreased venous return. This process can be seen in patients intubated during COPD or asthma exacerbations or patients ventilated with very high respiratory rates (e.g., as compensation for a severe metabolic acidosis), which are associated with decreased exhalation time.

Miscellaneous Hazards

Mechanical problems are a constant hazard. They include power failure, microprocessor malfunctions, broken connections, and kinking of tubes. Apnea alarms are available to warn of these dangers, but skilled care by the intensive care team is essential.

Pneumothorax can occur, especially if PEEP and/or unusually large tidal volumes are used. *Interstitial emphysema* may develop if the lung is overdistended. The air escapes from ruptured alveoli, tracks along the perivascular and peribronchial interstitium (see Figure 6.1), and may enter the mediastinum and the subcutaneous tissue of the neck and chest wall.

Excessive tidal volumes can also cause *ventilator-induced lung injury* due to repetitive overstretching of the alveoli. Careful attention to ensure patients do not receive tidal volumes more than 8 to 10 mL/kg of their ideal body weight is critical for preventing this issue.

Ventilator-associated pneumonia can develop in patients who remain on mechanical ventilation for more than a short period. *Cardiac arrhythmias* may be caused by rapid swings in pH and hypoxemia. There is also an increased incidence of *gastrointestinal bleeding* in these patients who are not receiving enteral nutrition while being ventilated.

Several complications are associated with endotracheal and tracheostomy tubes. Ulceration of the larynx or the trachea is sometimes seen, particularly if the inflated cuff exerts undue pressure on the mucosa. This can lead to scarring and tracheal stenosis, damage to the cartilaginous rings in the trachea, and development of a tracheoesophageal fistula. The use of large-volume, low-pressure cuffs has reduced the incidence of these problems considerably. Care must be taken with the placement of an endotracheal tube to avoid inadvertent placement of the distal end of the tube in the right main bronchus, which can cause atelectasis of the left lung and often the right upper lobe.

KEY CONCEPTS

1. Mechanical ventilation has a major role in treating patients with respiratory failure. Ventilatory support can be delivered invasively through an endotracheal tube or a tracheostomy tube or noninvasively through a tight-fitting mask.

2. Most ventilators support patients through positive-pressure ventilation. Tank, or negative pressure, ventilators are now seldom used except for patients with long-term neuromuscular disease.

3. There are multiple modes for delivering positive-pressure ventilation. These modes are frequently combined with positive end-expiratory pressure (PEEP) to improve oxygenation in patients with severe hypoxemia.

4. Mechanical ventilation, especially when used with an increased oxygen concentration and PEEP, typically increases the arterial P_{O_2} and reduces the P_{CO_2}. However, it can reduce venous return and may cause pneumothorax and other complications.

CLINICAL VIGNETTE

A 54-year-old woman presents to the Emergency Department with 2 days of dyspnea, fever, productive cough, and pleuritic right-sided chest pain. After a chest radiograph demonstrates a right lower lobe opacity, she is diagnosed with pneumonia and admitted to the hospital ward. Although she was started on appropriate antibiotic therapy, she develops increased difficulty with her breathing and hypoxemia and requires transfer to the ICU. Despite use of high-flow oxygen, she remains hypoxemic and requires intubation and initiation of invasive mechanical ventilation. A chest radiograph done following intubation now shows diffuse bilateral opacities. She is started on volume control ventilation with a tidal volume of 550 mL, a respiratory rate of 20, F_IO_2 1.0, and PEEP 5 cm H_2O. The following data were obtained before and 30 minutes following intubation:

Time Point	Blood Pressure (mm Hg)	Pa_{O_2} (mm Hg)	Pa_{CO_2} (mm Hg)
Preintubation	130/77	51	46
Postintubation	98/69	58	38

Questions

- How do you account for the observed change in her Pa_{CO_2} following intubation?
- What changes would you expect to occur in her dead space following intubation?
- What effect will the findings on chest radiography have on the pressure needed to inflate her lungs on inhalation?
- What intervention can you consider to improve her oxygenation?
- How do you account for the decrease in her blood pressure following intubation?

QUESTIONS

1. A 40-year-old man is receiving invasive mechanical ventilation for severe ARDS. He is ventilated using the volume control mode with a rate of 15 breaths per minute, tidal volume of 500 mL, and PEEP 5 cm H_2O. After increasing the F_IO_2 from 0.5 to 1.0, his Pa_{O_2} remained less than 60 mm Hg. Which of the following interventions is most appropriate to improve his oxygenation?
   A. Increase the tidal volume
   B. Increase the respiratory rate
   C. Increase the PEEP
   D. Increase the inspiratory flow rate
   E. Change to pressure control ventilation

2. A 66-year-old woman is intubated to prevent aspiration of blood after presenting with hemorrhagic shock due to an upper gastrointestinal bleeding. She is placed on volume control ventilation with an F_IO_2 of 0.5 and tidal volume of 450 mL. Following intubation, her blood pressure falls from 110/70 mm Hg to 85/50 mm Hg. On exam, she has equal breath sounds bilaterally and her trachea remains in the midline position. Which of the following is most likely responsible for the observed change in her blood pressure?
   A. Decrease in venous return
   B. Hypercarbia
   C. Placement of the endotracheal tube into the right mainstem bronchus
   D. Pneumothorax
   E. Resorption atelectasis

3. You are looking at the ventilator being used on a patient intubated for severe respiratory failure. The ventilator is set to deliver 10 breaths per minute, but the patient is receiving a total of 18 breaths per minute. With each breath, the pressure is increased 10 cm H_2O above the set PEEP and maintained at that level for 1 second. The volume delivered appears to vary over time. Which of the following modes is being used to ventilate the patient?

   A. Continuous positive airway pressure
   B. High-frequency oscillatory ventilation
   C. Pressure control
   D. Pressure support
   E. Volume control

4. A patient with paralyzed respiratory muscles but normal lungs is being treated by mechanical ventilation. In this patient, the arterial P_{CO_2} can be reduced without changing total ventilation by:

   A. Reducing the FRC
   B. Increasing the tidal volume
   C. Increasing the respiratory frequency
   D. Reducing the resistance of the airways
   E. Adding oxygen to the inspired gas

5. Which of the following patients is most appropriate for use of noninvasive positive-pressure ventilation?

   A. Acute respiratory distress syndrome
   B. Chronic obstructive pulmonary disease exacerbation
   C. Acute alteration in mental status with excessive airway secretions
   D. Guillain-Barré syndrome with long duration of need for respiratory support
   E. Large laryngeal mass occluding the opening to the trachea

6. In the treatment of a patient with ARDS by mechanical ventilation, the addition of PEEP typically results in:

   A. Reduced arterial P_{O_2}
   B. Reduced FRC
   C. Increased shunt
   D. Reduced physiologic dead space
   E. Tendency to reduce venous return to the thorax

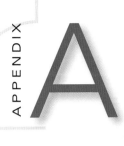

SYMBOLS, UNITS, AND NORMAL VALUES

SYMBOLS

Primary

C	Concentration of gas in blood
F	Fractional concentration in dry gas
P	Pressure or partial pressure
Q	Volume of blood
$\dot{Q}$	Volume of blood per unit time
R	Respiratory exchange ratio
S	Saturation of hemoglobin with O_2
V	Volume of gas
$\dot{V}$	Volume of gas per unit time

Secondary Symbols for Gas Phase

A	Alveolar
B	Barometric
D	Dead space
E	Expired
I	Inspired
L	Lung
T	Tidal

Secondary Symbols for Blood Phase

a	arterial
c	capillary
c′	end-capillary
i	ideal
v	venous
$\bar{v}$	mixed venous

Examples

O_2 concentration in arterial blood Ca_{O_2}
Fractional concentration of N_2 in expired gas $F_{E_{N_2}}$
Partial pressure of O_2 in mixed venous blood $P\bar{v}_{O_2}$

UNITS

Traditional metric units are used in this book. Pressures are given in mm Hg; the torr is an almost identical unit.

In Europe, SI (Système International) units are now commonly used. Most of them are familiar, but the kilopascal, the unit of pressure, is confusing at first. One kilopascal = 7.5 mm Hg (approximately).

Conversion of Gas Volumes to BTPS

Lung volumes, including FEV and FVC, are conventionally expressed at body temperature (37°C), ambient pressure, and saturated with water vapor (BTPS). To convert volumes measured in a spirometer at ambient temperature (t), pressure, saturated (ATPS) to BTPS,

$$\frac{310}{273+t} \cdot \frac{P_B - P_{H_2O}(t)}{P_B - 47}$$

In practice, tables are available for this conversion.

The derivation of this equation and all the other equations is given in the companion volume (*West's Respiratory Physiology: The Essentials*. 10th ed. p. 200).

REFERENCE VALUES

Reference Values for Lung Function Tests

Normal values depend on age, gender, height, weight, and ethnic origin. This is a complex subject; for a detailed discussion, see pages 333–365 of Cotes JE, Chinn DJ, Miller MR. *Lung Function*. 6th ed. Oxford, UK: Blackwell, 2006. Reference values for some common tests are shown in **Table A.1**. There is evidence that people are becoming healthier and that lung function is improving.

Table A.1	Example of Reference Values for Common Pulmonary Function Tests in White Nonsmoking Adults in the United States	
	Men	**Women**
TLC (L)	7.95 St* + 0.003 A† − 7.33 (0.79)‡	5.90 St − 4.54 (0.54)
FVC (L)	7.74 St − 0.021 A − 7.75 (0.51)	4.14 St − 0.023 A − 2.20 (0.44)
RV (L)	2.16 St + 0.021 A − 2.84 (0.37)	1.97 St + 0.020 A − 2.42 (0.38)
FRC (L)	4.72 St + 0.009 A − 5.29 (0.72)	3.60 St + 0.003 A − 3.18 (0.52)
RV/TLC (%)	0.309 A + 14.1 (4.38)	0.416 A + 14.35 (5.46)
FEV_1 (L)	5.66 St − 0.023 A − 4.91 (0.41)	2.68 St − 0.025 A − 0.38 (0.33)
FEV_1/FVC (%)	110.2 − 13.1 St − 0.15 A (5.58)	124.4 − 21.4 St − 0.15 A (6.75)
$FEF_{25-75\%}$ (L·s^{-1})	5.79 St − 0.036 A − 4.52 (1.08)	3.00 St − 0.031 A − 0.41 (0.85)
$MEF_{50\% FVC}$ (L·s^{-1})	6.84 St − 0.037 A − 5.54 (1.29)	3.21 St − 0.024 A − 0.44 (0.98)
$MEF_{25\% FVC}$ (L·s^{-1})	3.10 St − 0.023 A − 2.48 (0.69)	1.74 St − 0.025 A − 0.18 (0.66)
DI (mL·min^{-1} ·mm Hg^{-1})	16.4 St − 0.229 A + 12.9 (4.84)	16.0 St − 0.111 A + 2.24 (3.95)
DI/V_A	10.09 − 2.24 St − 0.031 A (0.73)	8.33 − 1.81 St − 0.016 A (0.80)

*St is stature (height) (m).
†A is age (years).
‡Standard deviation is in parentheses.
From Cotes JE, Chinn DJ, Miller MR. *Lung Function*. 6th ed. Oxford, UK: Blackwell, 2006.

FURTHER READING

Courtney Broaddus V, Mason RJ, Ernst JD, King TE, Lazarus SC, Murray JF, Nadel JA, Slutsky AS, Gotway MB. *Murray and Nadel's Textbook of Respiratory Medicine*. 6th ed. Philadelphia, PA: Saunders Elsevier, 2015.

Crystal RG, West JB, Weibel ER, Barnes PJ. *The Lung: Scientific Foundations*. 2nd ed. Philadelphia, PA: Lippincott-Raven, 1997.

Grippi MA, Elias JA, Fishman JA, Kotloff RM, Pack AI, Senior RM. *Fishman's Pulmonary Diseases and Disorders*. 5th ed. New York, NY: McGraw-Hill Education, 2015.

Kumar V, Abbas AK, Aster JC. *Robbins and Cotran Pathologic Basis of Disease*. 9th ed. Philadelphia, PA: Saunders Elsevier, 2014.

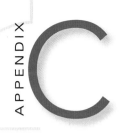
ANSWERS TO THE END-OF-CHAPTER QUESTIONS

CHAPTER 1

Question 1. A is correct. Fixed upper airway obstruction reduces both the inspiratory and expiratory flow rates. The other choices are incorrect. The response to bronchodilator drugs is best measured during expiration, and the inspiratory flow–volume curve is not useful for differentiating between chronic bronchitis and emphysema, detecting resistance in small airways, or detecting fatigue of the diaphragm.

Question 2. B is correct. The slope of phase 3 is increased in chronic bronchitis because poorly ventilated units receive less oxygen during the inspiration and also tend to empty last. The other choices are incorrect. The single breath nitrogen test is abnormal in mild COPD; poorly ventilated units tend to empty last; in normal subjects, the last expired gas comes from the upper part of the lung; and during the test, the expiratory flow rate should be limited to $0.5 \ L \cdot s^{-1}$.

Question 3. C is correct. The closing volume is raised when there is an increase in resistance of the small, peripheral airways because they then close at an abnormally high volume. The other choices are incorrect. Closing volume increases with age, it is poorly reproducible, it is most informative in patients with relatively mild lung disease, and it is raised in mild COPD.

Question 4. B is correct. This woman has airflow obstruction on spirometry as evidenced by the low FEV_1/FVC ratio. This develops due to dynamic compression of the airways. Lung compliance is increased in emphysema, while radial traction on the airways is decreased due to the loss of elastic recoil, and the blood–gas barrier has normal thickness. The diaphragm is not weak in these patients, although contractile efficiency may be diminished due to hyperinflation.

Question 5. D is correct. Although smokers commonly develop obstructive lung disease, the spirometry is consistent with a restrictive process, such as pulmonary fibrosis. Asthma, chronic bronchitis, and chronic obstructive pulmonary disease would cause airflow obstruction, while pulmonary hypertension is typically associated with normal spirometry.

Question 6. E is correct. Better effort on spirometry leads to increased peak expiratory flow but will not change flow at end-exhalation when flow is limited by dynamic airway compression. Vital capacity would be expected to increase with better effort, while flattening of the expiratory and inspiratory limbs of the flow–volume loops occurs with various forms of upper airway obstruction rather than as a function of patient effort.

Question 7. D is correct. The flow–volume loop has a "scooped out" appearance often seen in patients with airflow obstruction. Of the items on the list of choices, increased airway secretions is the one that could cause airflow obstruction by increasing airway resistance. Fibrosis of the lung parenchyma and increased elastic recoil would be associated with normal flows but decreased vital capacity. Increased radial traction on the airways would improve rather than limit airflow, while the number of pulmonary capillaries has no effect on spirometry.

CHAPTER 2

Question 1. D is correct. An increased 2,3-DPG concentration allows more oxygen to be unloaded because it reduces the oxygen affinity of hemoglobin, that is, it shifts the dissociation curve to the right. All the other choices increase the oxygen affinity.

Question 2. A is correct. Since the P_{CO_2} is raised and the pH is reduced, there is a respiratory acidosis. However, the pH of 7.20 is too low to be explained by the P_{CO_2} of 50 mm Hg, and so there must be a concomitant metabolic acidosis. This is common after surgery because a reduced blood flow and the resulting tissue hypoxia in some areas result in the production of lactic acid.

Question 3. D is correct. The only mechanism of hypoxemia that prevents the arterial P_{O_2} from reaching the expected level if 100% oxygen is inspired is shunt. In all the other mechanisms, the P_{O_2} will rise to the expected level, although this may take a long time with severe ventilation–perfusion inequality.

Question 4. E is correct. Exercise at high altitude is one of the few situations where oxygen transfer is diffusion limited in the normal lung. In none of the other four choices is gas transfer limited by diffusion, and therefore, doubling the diffusing capacity will have no effect.

Question 5. E is correct. The reduced pH indicates an acidosis, but the fact that the P_{CO_2} is reduced means that this cannot be respiratory. Furthermore, the bicarbonate concentration of 25 mmol·L^{-1} is normal or slightly high, and this rules out a metabolic acidosis. Therefore, there must be a laboratory error.

Question 6. D is correct. The patient's FEV$_1$/FVC ratio and TLC are normal while the diffusion capacity for carbon monoxide is decreased. This can occur due to anemia as the decreased hemoglobin concentration leads to decreased uptake of carbon monoxide across the alveolar–capillary barrier during the test. Asthma and chronic obstructive pulmonary disease cause reductions in the FEV_1/FVC ratio while idiopathic pulmonary fibrosis decreases TLC and sarcoidosis has variable effects on pulmonary function testing.

Question 7. B is correct. The arterial blood gas demonstrates a primary metabolic acidosis with respiratory compensation, which can be seen in diabetic ketoacidosis. Chronic obstructive pulmonary disease exacerbation, morbid obesity, and opiate overdoses would be associated with primary respiratory acidosis, while severe vomiting would cause a primary metabolic alkalosis.

Question 8. B is correct. With ascent to high altitude, the pressure gradient for diffusion across the alveolar–capillary barrier is diminished. This will slow the rate of rise of the P_{O_2} in the pulmonary capillaries. Individuals hyperventilate following ascent due to increased peripheral chemoreceptor stimulation. This leads to a respiratory rather than a metabolic alkalosis. The shunt fraction does not change following ascent, while the diffusion capacity for carbon monoxide might actually increase because increased cardiac output leads to recruitment and distention of capillaries.

Question 9. A is correct. Movement from condition A to condition B is associated with an increase in the $P_{A_{O_2}}$ and decrease in the $P_{A_{CO_2}}$, changes consistent with hyperventilation. Anxiety is the only item in the list of choices that causes hyperventilation. The other items all cause hypoventilation.

Question 10. D is correct. The patient has hypoxemia and an increased alveolar–arterial oxygen difference (39 mm Hg). This is seen with ventilation–perfusion inequality. It can also be seen in shunt, but this was not an answer choice. Hypoventilation is not present given the normal Pa_{CO_2}, while low $P_{I_{O_2}}$ is ruled out because she is at sea level. Diffusion impairment does not cause hypoxemia in individuals at rest at sea level.

CHAPTER 3

Question 1. D is correct. The alveoli at the top of the lungs are larger than those at the base because the lung tissue is distorted by its weight (see Figure 3.4). All the other choices are incorrect because they refer to variables that are reduced at the apex of the lung.

Question 2. B is correct. β_2-Agonists reduce airway resistance in asthma and indeed are some of the most valuable medications. The other choices are incorrect. Airway resistance is decreased at high lung volumes. Destruction of alveolar walls does not typically occur in asthma. Airway resistance is increased by obstructions in the airways, for example, retained secretions. Airway resistance is also increased by hypertrophy of bronchial smooth muscle, so we can expect loss of some of the muscle to decrease resistance.

Question 3. A is correct. A patient with mitral stenosis tends to have a reduced cardiac output and therefore impaired perfusion of skeletal muscle at a relatively low level of exercise. The result will be an increased blood lactate level, which stimulates ventilation, and therefore washes out CO_2 and causes the respiratory exchange ratio to rise about 1. The other choices are incorrect. The high respiratory exchange ratio is caused by an abnormally high ventilation, cardiac output is abnormally low, and lung compliance and diffusing capacity are not relevant.

Question 4. E is correct. The ventilation–perfusion scan shows an area of lung that receives ventilation but no perfusion. This finding occurs in pulmonary embolism. Asthma and chronic obstructive pulmonary disease exacerbations would cause heterogeneity on the ventilation images but not the perfusion images, while pneumothorax might show impaired ventilation and perfusion in the same region. Myocardial infarction would not affect the ventilation or perfusion images.

Question 5. E is correct. Functional residual capacity is determined by the balance of the recoil of the lung and chest wall. In a patient with evidence of obstructive lung disease due to emphysema, the functional residual capacity would increase due to decreased lung recoil. Airway resistance, total lung capacity, and lung compliance are often increased in these patients, while the diffusion capacity for carbon monoxide is decreased.

Question 6. B is correct. Plethysmography measures all the gas in the lung, while the helium dilution technique "sees" only those regions of the lung that communicate with the mouth. Therefore, regions behind closed airways result in a higher value for the plethysmographic than for the dilution procedure. This phenomenon can be seen in patients with chronic obstructive lung disease but not the other diseases on the list.

CHAPTER 4

Question 1. B is correct. Centriacinar emphysema initially occurs in the upper part of the lung see Figure 4.5A. The other choices are incorrect. The emphysema caused by α_1-antitrypsin deficiency often preferentially affects the base of the lung. The other choices do not have a typical regional distribution.

Question 2. C is correct. Patients with a type A presentation tend to have large increase in lung compliance. The other choices are incorrect. These patients have less cough productive of sputum, larger lung volumes, less hypoxemia, and a lesser tendency to develop cor pulmonale. Some people might question whether C is always correct, but the other options are clearly incorrect, so C is the best answer.

Question 3. E is correct. The FRC often falls when a patient with asthma is treated with a bronchodilator. However, more important is that all the other options are clearly incorrect. All these measurements from a forced expiration typically increase following administration of a bronchodilator.

Question 4. C is correct. The information provided indicates that this patient has chronic obstructive pulmonary disease, which is associated with decreased vascular markings on chest radiography. The retrosternal airspace is typically enlarged in these patients. Bilateral hilar lymphadenopathy is associated with sarcoidosis and lymphoma, while reticular opacities are seen with diffuse pulmonary fibrosis, and bilateral opacities are seen in pulmonary edema.

Question 5. D is correct. This young woman has asthma that is not under adequate control. Because asthma is an inflammatory disorder, she should begin daily use of an inhaled corticosteroid. Many physicians believe that inhaled long-acting β_2-agonists should not be used as the primary controller medication unless a patient is already on inhaled steroids. The other medications listed would not be appropriate as the first-line controller medication.

Question 6. B is correct. While this patient is a smoker and has airflow obstruction, he is younger than expected for a diagnosis of chronic obstructive pulmonary disease. His age, limited smoking history, and the fact that the lucent areas of his lung on chest imaging are primarily at his lung bases suggest he has α_1-antitrypsin deficiency, which causes a panacinar emphysema. Patients who present this early are usually homozygous for the Z-gene and often develop extrapulmonary disease. The emphysema is bilateral, and treatment is available with replacement of α_1-antitrypsin.

Question 7. E is correct. This woman has chronic obstructive pulmonary disease. Air-trapping commonly leads to an increased residual volume in these patients. Functional residual capacity is increased due to decreased lung recoil, while diffusion capacity for carbon monoxide is decreased due to the loss of surface area for gas exchange. The total lung capacity and RV/TLC ratio are often increased due to air-trapping and increased lung compliance.

Question 8. E is correct. Ventilation–perfusion inequality is the predominant cause of hypoxemia in patients with acute severe asthma. Shunt can occur when there is mucous plugging of the airways, and this may contribute to her hypoxemia. She is not hypoventilating at this time. Hyperventilation would actually increase the P_{aO_2} in the absence of ventilation–perfusion inequality. Diffusion impairment is not a cause of hypoxemia in these patients.

CHAPTER 5

Question 1. C is correct. The clinical and radiographic findings in this case are consistent with diffuse interstitial pulmonary fibrosis. Because of the increased radial traction on the airways, the FEV_1/FVC ratio is typically increased. However, the FEV_1, FVC, and TLC are reduced. Airway resistance when related to lung volume is also reduced.

Question 2. A is correct. The arterial P_{O_2} of a patient with diffuse interstitial pulmonary fibrosis typically falls during exercise. The other choices are incorrect. The hypoxemia is chiefly caused by ventilation–perfusion inequality, not by diffusion impairment, though this can contribute to the hypoxemia during exercise. The diffusing capacity typically increases little on exercise. Carbon dioxide retention is not a feature. The hypoxemia worsens during exercise and is typically associated with an abnormally small increase in cardiac output.

Question 3. D is correct. The increased radial traction on the airways explains the higher flow rate in relation to lung volume compared with a normal subject. The other choices are incorrect. The high flow rate is not related to the mechanical advantage of the expiratory muscles, the airways have a larger diameter if anything, and dynamic compression of the airways is less likely than in a normal subject. Airway resistance is decreased.

Question 4. A is correct. Amyotrophic lateral sclerosis (ALS) and idiopathic pulmonary fibrosis can both cause restrictive pathophysiology. Because pulmonary fibrosis thickens the blood-gas barrier and obliterates some capillaries, that patient would have a decreased diffusion capacity for carbon monoxide, whereas the lung parenchyma, surface area for gas exchange, and diffusion capacity would be normal in the ALS patient. The two patients will have similar findings with regard to the FEV_1, FEV_1/FVC ratio, FVC, and total lung capacity.

Question 5. D is correct. This woman has evidence of tension pneumothorax probably due to rupture of a bleb or bullae related to her chronic obstructive pulmonary disease. This is a medical emergency and should be treated with urgent needle decompression of the affected side. None of the other diagnostic tests or interventions would be appropriate.

Question 6. D is correct. The clinical and radiographic information in this case indicates that this patient likely has diffuse interstitial fibrosis. On pulmonary function testing, these patients demonstrate decreased FEV_1, FVC, TLC, and DLCO. The FEV_1/FVC ratio is normal and, in some cases, increased.

Question 7. C is correct. The finding of noncaseating granulomas in a patient with bilateral hilar lymphadenopathy is consistent with a diagnosis of sarcoidosis. Because he is asymptomatic with a normal examination, he will likely have normal pulmonary function. Spontaneous remission is commonly seen with his form of the disease. While he is at risk for involvement of other organs, he will not necessarily develop pulmonary fibrosis without treatment. In the absence of severe lung disease, he would be expected to have a normal arterial P_{CO_2}.

CHAPTER 6

Question 1. C is correct. If the colloid osmotic pressure of the blood is reduced, there is less of a tendency for fluid to move into the capillaries. The other choices are incorrect. The permeability of the alveolar epithelial cells is not relevant to fluid movement between the capillary lumen and the interstitium of the alveolar wall. A reduced capillary hydrostatic pressure, an increased hydrostatic pressure in the interstitial space, and a reduced colloid osmotic pressure of the interstitial fluid will all tend to move fluid from the interstitium into the capillary lumen.

Question 2. A is correct. In early interstitial edema, fluid moves from the capillary lumen into the interstitium of the thick side of the capillary wall. There is no movement of fluid into the thin side. The other choices are incorrect. The alveolar epithelium has a very low permeability for water, the strength of the barrier on the thin side is mainly attributable to the type IV collagen in the extracellular matrix, a small amount of protein normally crosses the capillary endothelium, and water is actively transported out of the alveolar spaces by alveolar epithelial cells.

Question 3. E is correct. In early interstitial edema, cuffs of fluid collect around the small pulmonary arteries and veins. The other choices are incorrect. As stated in the answer to Question 2 above, fluid from the capillary lumen does not enter the thin side of the blood–gas barrier. In the early stages of pulmonary edema, there is an increase in lung lymph flow. However, fluid does not enter the alveoli in interstitial edema. In early interstitial edema, the hydrostatic pressure in the interstitium rises as fluid enters it, and this tends to inhibit further movement of fluid from the capillary lumen to the interstitium.

Question 4. A is correct. Interstitial pulmonary edema is difficult to detect, but short, linear, horizontal markings near the pleural surface known as "septal lines" can be seen on a chest radiograph. The other choices are incorrect. Lung compliance may fall, lymph flow from the lung increases, there is little if any impairment of gas exchange and certainly no severe hypoxemia, and fluffy shadowing occurs on the chest radiograph in alveolar edema but not interstitial edema.

Question 5. C is correct. Blood passing through regions of the lung with alveolar edema constitutes a shunt, and therefore, the arterial PO_2 does not rise to the expected level while breathing 100% oxygen. The other choices are incorrect. Lung compliance is reduced, airway resistance is increased because some airways are blocked with fluid, respiration is typically shallow and rapid, but the edema does not cause chest pain.

Question 6. B is correct. The embolized areas do not eliminate CO_2, and therefore, the physiologic dead space is increased. The other choices are incorrect. CO_2 retention is not typical; pulmonary hypertension, not hypotension, occurs; rhonchi do not typically occur; cardiac output often falls.

Question 7. B is correct. The sudden onset of dyspnea and chest pain following a period of prolonged immobility as well as the finding of asymmetric leg edema on exam raises concern for pulmonary embolism. The most appropriate diagnostic test is a contrast-enhanced CT scan of the chest. Pulmonary angiography is the gold standard for diagnosis of pulmonary embolism but is very invasive and would not be done before a CT scan. The other choices would not yield the correct diagnosis in this case.

Question 8. B is correct. This patient has elevated pulmonary artery pressure in the setting of pulmonary edema due to left heart failure. Left ventricular failure leads to increased left ventricular end-diastolic and left atrial pressure, which contributes to increased pulmonary artery pressure. Without other evidence of sarcoidosis, granulomatous inflammation of the arterioles would not be expected. Increased pulmonary blood flow occurs with ventricular septal defects or patent ductus arteriosus but would not be expected in left ventricular failure. Her history is not consistent with either idiopathic pulmonary arterial hypertension, which would cause structural changes in the arterioles, or recurrent thromboembolism.

Question 9. E is correct. This individual likely has high-altitude pulmonary edema (HAPE), which develops as a result of exaggerated hypoxic pulmonary vasoconstriction. The arteriolar constriction is uneven and, as a result, regions of the capillary bed that are not protected from the high pressure and develop the ultrastructural changes of stress failure. Left ventricular function and, therefore, left atrial pressure are normal in HAPE, while colloid osmotic pressure and interstitial pressure are unaffected. Endotoxin-mediated increases in capillary permeability are seen in sepsis rather than at high altitude.

Question 10. C is correct. This patient with very severe COPD is now presenting with signs of cor pulmonale, including increased jugular venous distention, weight gain, and bilateral leg edema and characteristic changes on electrocardiography. The most appropriate test to confirm this diagnosis would be echocardiography. Since he is known to have COPD, spirometry would not provide further useful information. Duplex ultrasonography and contrast-enhanced CT are not indicated, as the suspicion for venous thromboembolism is low. Bronchoscopy would not be helpful in the evaluation of cor pulmonale.

CHAPTER 7

Question 1. D is correct. Nitrogen oxides in smog cause inflammation of the upper respiratory tract and are probably a factor in the development of chronic bronchitis. The other choices are incorrect. Ozone is not mainly produced by automobile engines but by the action of sunlight on hydrocarbons and nitrogen oxides in the atmosphere. The main cause of sulfur oxides is burning fossil fuel that contains sulfur. Scrubbing fuel gases is effective in removing particles but is expensive.

Question 2. B is correct. Heavy cigarette smokers can have up to 10% of their hemoglobin bound to carbon monoxide, and there is evidence that this can impair cognitive skills. The other choices are incorrect. Inhaled smoke contains substantial amounts of carbon monoxide. Nicotine is highly addictive. Smoking is an important risk factor in coronary heart disease, and the concentration of pollutants in inhaled cigarette smoke is typically higher than that in smog.

Question 3. E is correct. If a miner breathes through his nose, most of the larger particles will be trapped there. The other choices are incorrect. Coughing can help to remove particles but does not prevent their deposition. Exercise increases pulmonary ventilation and therefore increases deposition. Very small dust particles are deposited by sedimentation or diffusion, and rapid deep breathing increases deposition.

Question 4. E is correct. The mucous film is altered in some diseases such as asthma, where it becomes tenacious and difficult for the cilia to move. The other choices are incorrect. Although goblet cells in the airway epithelium produce some mucus, most of it comes from the seromucous glands in the airway wall. Trapped particles move much more rapidly in the trachea than in the peripheral airways. Normal clearance is complete in about a day or so, and cilia typically beat around 20 times per second.

Question 5. D is correct. Non–small cell bronchial carcinomas are very common. The other choices are incorrect. Lung cancer is now a more common cause of death than breast cancer in women in the United States; the carcinogenic agents in cigarette smoke, loosely described as tars, have not been fully identified; pulmonary function tests are not useful in the early detection of the disease, and some early carcinomas are not visible on the chest radiograph.

Question 6. A is correct. Many features of this patient's case suggest that he has diffuse pulmonary fibrosis. Given that he worked with insulation in the shipyards and has calcified pleural plaques on his chest radiograph, this is most likely due to asbestosis. His spirometry is not consistent with chronic obstructive pulmonary disease, and his chest radiograph and exposure history are not compatible with berylliosis, coal-worker's pneumoconiosis, or silicosis.

Question 7. B is correct. The diagnosis of pneumocystis pneumonia should always prompt evaluation for underlying immunosuppression, in particular human immunodeficiency virus (HIV) as it is uncommon in immunocompetent individuals. Sweat chloride testing is used to evaluate for cystic fibrosis. HIV-positive patients are at increased risk for TB, but skin testing would not be helpful in this situation. Spirometry and echocardiography would not be useful.

Question 8. C is correct. Large particles (greater than 20 μm in diameter) are very likely to be removed by the nose or impact the airway mucosa in the nasopharynx. Medium size particles (1 to 5 μm) will deposit by sedimentation in the terminal and respiratory bronchioles, while very small particles (less than 0.1 μm in diameter) may deposit by diffusion in the small airways and alveoli.

Question 9. A is correct. In pneumonia, the lung affected by the disease is not ventilated and, if it is perfused, the resulting shunt can cause hypoxemia. Patients with pneumonia usually recover with no residual pathology. Carbon dioxide retention is unlikely in most patients because of increased ventilation to other parts of the lung. Some common bacterial causes of pneumonia such as *Legionella* are difficult to grow on routine culture media while blood flow in the affected area is often decreased due, in part, to hypoxic pulmonary vasoconstriction.

Question 10. B is correct. Male cystic fibrosis patients are usually infertile due to defects in sperm transport. Mucociliary dysfunction is a major source of problems in these patients who often have disease in other organs including the pancreas and liver. Patients require lifelong treatment of their disease, but with effective care can now survive into their fourth decade of life or more.

CHAPTER 8

Question 1. B is correct. Patients with severe COPD and CO_2 retention (this patient's P_{CO_2} was 50 mm Hg) often have their ventilation partly driven by the low arterial P_{O_2}. If they are treated with 100% oxygen, this drive to ventilation is removed, and they may decrease their ventilation with a corresponding increase in P_{CO_2}. Changes in ventilation–perfusion matching due to decreased hypoxic pulmonary vasoconstriction also contribute. The other choices are incorrect. Administering oxygen does not increase airway resistance or depress cardiac output. Choices D and E are irrelevant.

Question 2. A is correct. An exacerbation of chronic obstructive pulmonary disease can cause an increase in arterial P_{CO_2} and therefore respiratory acidosis. The other choices are incorrect. Mechanical ventilation and administration of antibiotics will reduce the tendency to CO_2 retention. Renal retention of bicarbonate will reduce the acidosis by metabolic compensation.

Question 3. C is correct. A patient with ARDS typically has severe hypoxemia caused by extensive ventilation–perfusion inequality, including blood flow through unventilated lung (shunt). The other choices are incorrect. Lung compliance and FRC are typically decreased, and a large shunt often occurs. Despite the severe ventilation–perfusion inequality, some patients have a low or normal $P_{a_{CO_2}}$.

Question 4. E is correct. The development of hypoxemic respiratory failure with diffuse opacities shortly after premature birth usually results from the infant respiratory distress syndrome due to insufficient pulmonary surfactant. In addition to supportive care, appropriate treatment includes administration of surfactant by the inhalational route. Bronchodilators would not be useful in this situation since the pathophysiology is related to extensive alveolar atelectasis. Diuretics and digoxin would also not be of use as the infant is not in heart failure.

Question 5. B is correct. An acute exacerbation of chronic obstructive pulmonary disease in a patient with severe COPD typically causes worsening of the ventilation–perfusion relationships. The other choices are incorrect. The COPD exacerbation increases the airway resistance, the arterial pH typically falls because of the respiratory acidosis, and an increase in the alveolar–arterial P_{O_2} difference is usual.

CHAPTER 9

Question 1. E is correct. Fifty percent oxygen raises the inspired P_{O_2} to about 350 mm Hg from its normal value of about 150 mm Hg. Therefore, if the P_{CO_2} does not change, we can expect the arterial P_{O_2} to rise by approximately 200 mm Hg. The other choices are incorrect.

Question 2. D is correct. The arterial P_{O_2} will rise because of the oxygen dissolved in the nonshunted blood. However, it cannot possibly rise to 600 mm Hg because of the shunt. Therefore, the only possible correct choices are C and D. Figure 9.3 and the accompanying text shows that the increase will be more than 10 mm Hg. However, choosing between C and D is challenging.

Question 3. B is correct. The presence of carbon monoxide in blood increases the oxygen affinity of the hemoglobin. The other choices are incorrect. A patient with CO poisoning may have a normal arterial P_{O_2}, or even an increased P_{O_2} if they are receiving supplemental oxygen, but this would not affect the P_{50}. The other choices all cause an increase in the P_{50} of the blood.

Question 4. C is correct. The inspired oxygen concentration with nasal cannulas can change greatly depending on the pattern of breathing and whether the patient is partly breathing through his mouth. The other choices are incorrect. Most patients find cannulas more comfortable than masks, inspired oxygen concentrations of about 25% can be obtained, there is no interference with the patient talking, and in most patients, the P_{CO_2} does not tend to rise. Although this could happen in a patient with respiratory failure whose respiratory drive comes partly from the arterial hypoxemia, the increase in arterial P_{O_2} is usually not sufficient for this to occur.

Question 5. E is correct. The solubility of oxygen is 0.003 ml 100 ml blood^{-1} mm Hg^{-1}. A pressure of three atmospheres is equivalent to 2,280 mm Hg, so that with an inspired concentration of 100%, we can expect the inspired P_{O_2} to rise to more than 2,000 mm Hg. Therefore, the amount of dissolved oxygen will be approximately 6 mL/100 mL.

Question 6. C is correct. When high concentrations of oxygen are administered, lung units with low ventilation–perfusion ratios may deliver oxygen into the blood faster than it is entering them by ventilation. The units therefore collapse. The other choices are incorrect. Pulmonary surfactant is not affected. Oxygen toxicity can cause alveolar edema, but this is not the mechanism of the collapse. Interstitial edema may occur around small airways, but this is not the mechanism, nor are any inflammatory changes in small airways, if in fact they do occur.

Question 7. A is correct. The significant increase in Pa_{O_2} and Sp_{O_2} following supplemental oxygen administration decreases peripheral chemoreceptor stimulation, leading to decreased minute and alveolar ventilation and a rise in the Pa_{CO_2}. Because alveolar P_{O_2} increases with supplemental oxygen, ventilation–perfusion matching will worsen rather than improve. The hemoglobin–oxygen dissociation curve shifts to the right due to the increase Pa_{CO_2} but does not cause the hypercarbia. Increased hemoglobin–oxygen saturation decreases formation of carbamino groups on the hemoglobin chains, while the rise in Pa_{CO_2} causes a decrease in arterial pH.

CHAPTER 10

Question 1. C is correct. When the P_{O_2} does not rise significantly in patients with ARDS following a large increase in the $F_{I_{O_2}}$, the appropriate intervention is to increase the positive end-expiratory pressure (PEEP). Increasing the tidal volume and/or rate would increase minute ventilation, but this would likely not translate to an increase in the arterial P_{O_2} due to the severe ventilation–perfusion mismatch and shunt. Increasing the flow rate would prolong the expiratory phase but would not affect oxygenation, while changing to pressure control ventilation would also have no effect on oxygenation if the same $F_{I_{O_2}}$ and PEEP were used.

Question 2. A is correct. The patient's blood pressure likely fell due to a decrease in venous return that occurred with initiation of positive pressure ventilation. This was likely exacerbated by the fact that she was volume-depleted due to her hemorrhagic shock. Tension pneumothorax can cause hypotension, but this is unlikely given that she has bilateral breath sounds and her trachea is in the midline position. Hypercarbia, resorption atelectasis, and right mainstem intubation would not affect her blood pressure.

Question 3. C is correct. The description provided corresponds to the pressure control mode of mechanical ventilation. Pressure support also involves raising the inspiratory pressure a preset amount above the set PEEP, but there is no set respiratory rate and inspiratory pressure ceases when flow decreases sufficiently rather than after a prespecified time period. Volume control involves administering a preset volume rather than an inspiratory pressure. The ventilator does not change airway pressure during inhalation or exhalation in continuous positive airway pressure. High-frequency ventilation involves using very small tidal volumes (50 to 150 mL) at a very high frequency.

Question 4. B is correct. If the total ventilation is kept constant, the alveolar ventilation can be raised by increasing the tidal volume. This raises the ratio of alveolar ventilation to total ventilation, but of course reduces the respiratory frequency. The other choices are incorrect. Reducing the FRC will not directly affect ventilation, although it may result in atelectatic areas. Increasing the respiratory frequency necessarily means lowering the tidal volume and thus reducing the ratio of alveolar ventilation to total ventilation. Reducing the resistance of the airways, if that can be done, will not change alveolar ventilation. Finally, adding oxygen to the inspired gas also does not change alveolar ventilation.

Question 5. B is correct. Noninvasive positive pressure ventilation is appropriate for use in patients with exacerbations of chronic obstructive pulmonary diseases, as multiple studies have shown improved outcomes when it is used for this purpose. Noninvasive ventilation is not effective with severe hypoxemic respiratory failure, as in ARDS, and would be inappropriate for patients expected to need ventilatory support for a prolonged period of time or with excessive airway secretions and altered mental status. Ventilation through a tracheotomy would be the appropriate intervention for a patient with a mass occluding their upper airway.

Question 6. E is correct. Positive end-expiratory pressure (PEEP) tends to reduce venous return to the thorax because it increases intrathoracic pressure. The other choices are incorrect. Typically, the addition of PEEP increases the arterial P_{O_2}, increases the FRC, reduces shunt, but increases physiologic dead space.

ANSWERS TO QUESTIONS IN CLINICAL VIGNETTES

CHAPTER 1

The FEV_1 is decreased while the FVC is within the normal range. The decreased FEV_1/FVC ratio indicates that the patient has airflow obstruction. The FEV_1 improves by 0.2 liter (7% change), while the FVC is unchanged following administration of a short-acting bronchodilator, indicating that the patient does not meet criteria for a bronchodilator response (increase in FEV_1 or FVC by 200 mL and 12% from prebronchodilator values). The presence of airflow obstruction in a young individual typically raises concern for asthma, but the presence of flattening of both the inspiratory and expiratory limbs of the flow volume loop strongly suggests that the airflow obstruction is due to something other than asthma. In particular, this pattern is consistent with a fixed upper airway obstruction. This patient was subsequently sent for a CT scan of the chest, which demonstrated extensive lymphadenopathy compressing the intrathoracic trachea. Surgical biopsy later confirmed this was due to lymphoma.

CHAPTER 2

Spirometry performed in clinic 2 weeks ago demonstrates severe airflow obstruction with increased RV but no significant increase in TLC or bronchodilator response. In a patient with a long history of tobacco use, these findings are consistent with those seen in chronic obstructive pulmonary disease (COPD). Her increased dyspnea along with a change in the frequency of her cough and a change in the character of her sputum production suggest she has a COPD exacerbation. On exam, this typically causes diffuse expiratory wheezes, a prolonged expiratory phase, and hyperresonant lung fields. The decreased diffusion capacity for carbon monoxide indicates that the surface area for gas exchange is decreased. When this occurs in the setting of airflow obstruction, it suggests the patient has underlying emphysema.

The arterial blood gas demonstrates an acute respiratory acidosis, a common finding in COPD exacerbations. The increased Pa_{CO_2} and the increased alveolar–arterial oxygen difference (22 mm Hg for R = 0.8) are caused by increased ventilation–perfusion inequality. By raising airway pressure on inhalation, noninvasive ventilation through a tight-fitting mask will increase her total and alveolar ventilation and, as a result, decrease her Pa_{CO_2}.

CHAPTER 3

This patient has hypersensitivity pneumonitis due to her pet cockatiel. Her pulmonary function tests demonstrate restrictive pathophysiology. The decreased diffusion capacity for carbon monoxide indicates that the restriction is due to an intraparenchymal process. FRC, which is due to the balance between lung and chest recoil decreases due to increased lung recoil. RV will likely be low because lung compliance is reduced and the interstitial lung disease leads to increased radial traction on her airways, which allows more air to exit the lungs on exhalation. The compliance of her lungs will decrease as a result of her parenchymal process, causing the pressure–volume curve for her lungs to shift down and to the right and have a lower slope than in a normal individual. While airway resistance is increased in obstructive lung diseases, in a diffuse interstitial process, the airways are unaffected and resistance should be normal. In fact, if radial traction on the airways increases as a result of her disease, then airway resistance at any lung volume would be lower than in a normal individual. During a cardiopulmonary exercise test, her arterial P_{O_2} would be expected to decrease due to increased ventilation-perfusion mismatch and possibly some diffusion impairment. Mixed venous P_{O_2} also decreases in exercise due to reduced oxygen delivery, and this will also contribute to the development of hypoxemia in the setting of ventilation–perfusion inequality.

CHAPTER 4

This patient is having an acute asthma exacerbation. In such cases, the functional residual capacity and residual volume are increased compared to when a patient is in his or her normal healthy state. The hyperinflation seen on chest radiograph would fit with such findings. The increased RV is due to premature airway closure on exhalation, while the cause of the increased FRC is not fully understood. Even though patients with asthma exacerbations are having airflow obstruction on exhalation, they commonly report that they have difficulty with inhalation. This is because the airway closure and hyperinflation create a mechanical disadvantage. One particular problem is the flattening of the diaphragm, which impairs its contractile efficiency. Hypoxemia in these situations is primarily due to ventilation–perfusion inequality, although in severe cases, shunt may contribute if considerable mucous plugging of airways is present. Despite the fact that he is having significant difficulty breathing, the Pa_{CO_2} is typically low during an asthma exacerbation due to increased ventilation resulting from stimulation of the peripheral chemoreceptors by hypoxemia or stimulation of intrapulmonary receptors. The finding of a rising arterial P_{CO_2} during an asthma exacerbation is an ominous finding and suggests that the patient is developing respiratory failure due to ventilatory muscle fatigue and increasing ventilation–perfusion inequality. Treatment for an asthma exacerbation includes supplemental oxygen, systemic corticosteroids, and nebulized β_2-agonists. If he fails to improve and manifests evidence of respiratory failure, he may require intubation and mechanical ventilation.

CHAPTER 5

The finding of noncaseating granulomas on transbronchial biopsy indicates that this patient has sarcoidosis. In addition to bilateral hilar lymphadenopathy, her chest radiograph demonstrates diffuse bilateral reticular lung opacities. Based on this finding as well as the fact that her FEV_1 and FVC are reduced with a normal FEV_1/FVC ratio, she will likely have a restrictive pathophysiology and, therefore, a low TLC. We would also anticipate from the radiographic findings that the blood–gas barrier is thickened and that many capillaries are obliterated and, therefore, her DLCO will be low. Because of the changes in her lung parenchyma, her lung compliance will be low and, therefore, the pressure–volume curve will be shifted down and to the right with a lower slope than in a healthy individual. On arterial blood gas, she will either have normal acid–base status or a compensated respiratory alkalosis. The latter finding can develop if the patient has hyperventilation due to hypoxemia and subsequent stimulation of the peripheral chemoreceptors and/or stimulation of intrapulmonary receptors. If her parenchymal lung disease worsens significantly despite treatment, she may ultimately develop respiratory failure and progressive hypercarbia. This would lead to a compensated respiratory acidosis. With exercise, her Pa_{O_2} will likely decrease and the alveolar–arterial oxygen difference will widen as a result of increased ventilation–perfusion inequality due to the extensive parenchymal lung disease.

CHAPTER 6

The acute onset of chest pain, dyspnea, and hypoxemia following repair of pelvic or long-bone fractures should always raise concern for pulmonary embolism. The diagnosis was confirmed in this case by identification of a filling defect on the CT pulmonary angiogram. The major risk factor for pulmonary embolism in this case was vascular injury related to her pelvic fracture and its surgical repair. A lack of mobility following her operation may also have contributed. In such settings, unfractionated or low molecular weight heparin is often given on a prophylactic basis to prevent this problem. Echocardiography might show an elevation in pulmonary artery pressure due to obstruction to blood flow, but this depends on the size of the embolus. Small emboli will have little effect, but larger emboli are more likely to do so. Pulmonary embolism increases the physiologic dead space, but her arterial P_{CO_2} remained normal because she was able to increase her total ventilation. In some cases, the hypoxemia, severe pain, and anxiety following pulmonary embolism cause patients to raise their total ventilation even more, in which case, a low P_{CO_2} may be seen. Hypoxemia develops primarily as a result of ventilation–perfusion inequality that develops due to redistribution of blood flow to the nonembolized regions of the lung.

CHAPTER 7

This patient has cystic fibrosis, a multisystem disease that develops due to one of a variety of mutations affecting the cystic fibrosis transmembrane regulator (CFTR). These defects lead to alterations in sodium and chloride transport, which impair mucous clearance and leads to plugging of airways as well as ducts in other organs. Decreased mucociliary transport subsequently leads to persistent inflammation and infection in the airways, which, over time, contributes to the development of bronchiectasis and airflow obstruction. The tubular structures seen in the upper lung zones are dilated airways and are indicative of the presence of bronchiectasis. Increased airway secretions typically lead to evidence of airflow obstruction on pulmonary function testing including decreased $FEF_{25-75\%}$, increased RV/TLC ratio, and decreased FEV_1/FVC. While hyperinflation can lead to a high TLC, some patients eventually develop a mixed obstructive–restrictive defect as the TLC declines due to extensive scarring. Airway clearance measures such as regular exercise, chest physiotherapy, and other devices, as well as medications such as inhaled DNAase and hypertonic saline are critical for the long-term health of these patients as they help remove secretions from the airways and mitigate the ongoing inflammation and infection that contributes to disease progression. Even with effective treatment, some patients are prone to development of hemoptysis, as the ongoing inflammation can erode into the hypertrophied bronchial circulation feeding the airway mucosa. Because the bronchial circulation is perfused under systemic pressure, the volume of expectorated blood can reach life-threatening levels.

CHAPTER 8

This patient has developed the acute respiratory distress syndrome (ARDS) as a consequence of severe pancreatitis. She developed respiratory failure within 7 days of the pancreatitis, has severe hypoxemia with a low $P_{a_{O_2}}/F_{I_{O_2}}$ ratio, has diffuse bilateral opacities on chest imaging, and there is no evidence that this is related to left heart dysfunction. Due to the extensive injury to the lung, we would expect respiratory system compliance to be markedly reduced and the pressure–volume curve is shifted downward and to the right. One manifestation of this will be that the mechanical ventilator will require high pressures to inflate her lung with each breath. The functional residual capacity is decreased, likely due to exaggeration of surface tension forces by the alveolar edema and exudate. The fact that her $P_{a_{O_2}}$ is only 66 mm Hg while she is receiving 100% oxygen indicates that shunt is the primary cause of her hypoxemia. This is due to the fact that blood continues to flow by alveoli that are filled with edema and exudate and, as a result, do not receive any ventilation. Despite the severe ventilation–perfusion inequality and shunt, the P_{CO_2} may be normal or even low as it is with this patient. This is because the large volume of gas delivered to the alveoli is sufficient to keep the arterial

P_{CO_2} normal but not the arterial P_{O_2} in the presence of severe ventilation–perfusion inequality. Other patients do develop hypercarbia.

CHAPTER 9

This patient has a left lower lobe pneumonia associated with severe hypoxemia. The fact that Pa_{O_2} only increases from 55 to 62 mm Hg while breathing an F_1O_2 of 1.0 indicates that shunt is the primary cause of hypoxemia; blood continues to perfuse alveoli that are unventilated because they are filled with an inflammatory exudate. Fever causes a rightward shift in the hemoglobin–oxygen dissociation curve (increased P_{50}) such that any given Pa_{O_2}, the oxygen saturation is lower. If the cardiac output does not increase sufficiently to compensate for the decrease in saturation, tissue oxygen delivery will decrease. Coupled with the increase in oxygen consumption due to infection and fever, this decrease in oxygen delivery will lead to increased tissue oxygen extraction and a fall in the mixed venous oxygen content. This is a disadvantage from the standpoint of his arterial oxygenation as the oxygen-depleted mixed venous blood cannot pick up oxygen as it traverses the capillary network in the left lower lobe. When oxygenation does not improve despite a high inspired oxygen fraction on mechanical ventilation, positive end-expiratory pressure (PEEP) can be increased to address the hypoxemia (see Chapter 10). This is often not effective in focal processes such as lobar pneumonia, however. One other consideration for this patient would be to give him a blood transfusion, as improving his hemoglobin concentration would increase tissue oxygen delivery and raise the mixed venous oxygen content. In the setting of shunt, such improvements in mixed venous oxygen content can improve arterial oxygen content.

CHAPTER 10

This patient was intubated for respiratory failure due to severe pneumonia. The fact that she had an increased Pa_{CO_2} prior to intubation indicates that she had inadequate alveolar ventilation in addition to her severe hypoxemia. With initiation of volume control ventilation, which provides a guaranteed level of minute ventilation, she is now receiving sufficient alveolar ventilation to eliminate the carbon dioxide produced in her tissues and the Pa_{CO_2} decreases. Even though her alveolar ventilation increased, it does not increase by the same amount as total ventilation because mechanical ventilation increases both the alveolar and anatomic dead spaces. A factor here is that the increase in lung volume and application of PEEP increase radial traction on the airways increasing anatomic dead space. Increased airway pressure can also divert blood flow away from ventilated regions causing areas of high ventilation–perfusion ratio or even no perfusion at all.

Her chest radiograph following intubation revealed development of diffuse bilateral opacities, which, along with her severe hypoxemia, indicate she has developed ARDS as a complication of pneumonia. These opacities suggest that lung compliance is likely decreased. As a result, more pressure will be needed to inflate her lungs to the desired tidal volume than would be necessary to achieve the same volume in a person with normal lungs. Despite breathing an inspired oxygen concentration of 100%, her arterial P_{O_2} remains low. In such cases, it is appropriate to raise the PEEP above 5 cm H_2O. This will increase end-expiratory lung volume and prevent atelectasis and, as a result, improve gas exchange. While the patient's blood pressure may have decreased due to worsening of septic shock due to pneumonia, it may also be related to initiation of mechanical ventilation. Positive pressure ventilation increases intrathoracic pressure, which can decrease venous return and cardiac output, particularly when patients are volume depleted, as is often the case in sepsis.

INDEX

Note: Page numbers in *italics* indicate figures; and those followed by t indicate tables.

A

Absorption atelectasis, 199–201, *200*
Acid-base status
  Henderson-Hasselbalch equation, 34
  metabolic acidosis, 36
  metabolic alkalosis, 36
  respiratory acidosis, 34–35, *35*
  respiratory alkalosis, 36
Acidosis
  definition, 34
  metabolic, 36
  respiratory, 34–35, *35*
  respiratory failure, 177
Acinus, 63
Acute overwhelming lung disease, 178–179
Acute respiratory distress syndrome (ARDS), 216, 239, 241
  clinical features, 181–182
  mechanical ventilation, 218
  noninvasive mechanical ventilation, 207
  pathogenesis, 181
  pathology, 180–181, *180*
  PEEP, *211*, 213, 217, 218
  pulmonary function, 182–183
  respiratory failure, 174
β-Adrenergic agonist, 85
Aerosol deposition in lungs
  clearance mechanisms
    alveolar macrophages, 154–155
    mucociliary system, 153–154, *154*
  diffusion, 152
  impaction, 149, *150*
  sedimentation, 150–152, *150*, *151*
Airway closure, 14–15
Airway compression, 8–9
Airway conductance
  cigarette smoking effect, *48*
  elastic recoil pressure, airway obstruction, 75–76, *76*

Airway obstruction, 62, *62*
  bronchial, 91–92
  local, 91–92
Airway resistance
  asthma, 57, 89, 225
  bronchial asthma, 48, 89
  byssinosis, 157–158
  chronic bronchitis, 48
  COPD, 75
  dynamic compression of airways, 8, *9*, *10*
  edema, 129
  forced expiration, 7
  interpretation, 47–49
  management, 184
  measurement, 47
  tracheal obstruction, 49
Alkalosis
  metabolic, 36
  respiratory, 36
Alveolar dead space, 210
Alveolar edema, 123, *124*
Alveolar gas equation, 22, 30
Alveolar macrophages, 97, 154–155
Alveolar ventilation, 210
Alveolar ventilation equation, 22
Alveolar wall structure
  cell types
    epithelial cell, 97, *98*, *99*
    fibroblast, 99
    macrophage, 97
  interstitium, 99
Alveolar–arterial P_{O_2} difference, 29, 76
Amyotrophic lateral sclerosis (ALS), 118, 228
Anaerobic glycolysis, 175–176
Anaerobic threshold, 50
Anatomic dead space, 210
Ankylosing spondylitis, 115–116
Antibiotic therapy, 216
Anticholinergics, 86

Anti-IgE therapy, 87
α_1-Antitrypsin deficiency, 66, 67, 226
Arterial blood gas, 225
Arterial P_{CO_2}
  asthma, 91
  causes of, 32
  hypoventilation, 32–33
  measurement, 32
  mechanical ventilation, 210–213
  normal values, 32
  ventilation control, 80
  ventilation–perfusion inequality,
    33–34, *33*
Arterial pH
  acidosis, 34–36
  alkalosis, 36
  measurement, 34
Arterial P_{O_2}
  diffuse interstitial pulmonary fibrosis, 228
  hypoxemia (*see* Hypoxemia)
  measurement, 21
  normal values, 21–22, *21*
  oxygen unloading, 38
Arteriovenous malformation, pulmonary, 141
Asbestosis, 111
Asbestos-related diseases, 156–157
Asthma
  bronchoactive drugs
    β-adrenergic agonist, 85
    anticholinergics, 86
    cromolyn and nedocromil, 86–87
    FRC value, 94, 226–227
    inhaled corticosteroids, 86
    leukotriene receptor antagonists, 87
    5-lipoxygenase inhibitors, 87
    methylxanthines, 87
    omalizumab, 87
  clinical features, 84–85
  exacerbation, 237
  pathogenesis, 82–84, *83*
  pathology, 82, *83*
  pulmonary function
    gas exchange, 89–91, *89*, *90*
    ventilatory capacity and mechanics,
      87–89, *88*
Atelectasis, 199–201, *200*
Atmospheric pollutants
  carbon monoxide, 147
  cigarette smoke, 149
  hydrocarbons, 148
  nitrogen oxides, 148
  particulate matter, 148

  photochemical oxidants, 148
  sulfur oxides, 148
  in United States, 147
Auto-PEEP, 215

B

Bilateral hilar lymphadenopathy,
  noncaseating granulomas, 228
Blastomycosis, 162
Blood
  acid-base status, 34–36, *35*
  oxygen
    hemoglobin, 197
    hyperbaric, 197–198
    O_2 dissociation curve, 21–22, *21*
Blood stasis, 131
Blood–gas barrier
  edematous thickening, 129
  hypoxemia, 26
  in normal lung, 143, 228
  reduced diffusing capacity,
    37–38, 106
Blood-tissue gas exchange, 21–36
Body plethysmograph, 45, *48*
Boyle's law, 45
Breathing mechanics
  airway resistance
    interpretation, 47–49
    measurement, 47
  lung, elastic properties
    compliance, 46
    interpretation, 46–47, *48*
    measurement, 46, *46*
  uneven ventilation, 12–16
  ventilation (*see* Ventilation)
Bronchial carcinoma
  clinical features, 160
  incidence, 158
  non-small cell bronchial
    carcinomas, 231
  non–small-cell carcinoma, 159, 168
  pathogenesis, 158–159
  pulmonary function, 160
  small-cell carcinoma, 159
Bronchial obstruction, 91–92
Bronchial smooth muscle contraction, 48
Bronchiectasis, 163–164
Bronchoconstriction, 129
Bronchodilator, bronchial asthma, *88*
Byssinosis, 157–158

C

Carbon dioxide
  in arterial blood, 33–34, *33*
  retention, 197–198
  ventilatory response, 49
Carbon monoxide (CO)
  diffusing capacity
    reduced, 37–38
    single-breath method, 37, *37*
  hazards, 147
Cardiac arrhythmias, 215
Cardiac output
  oxygen delivery, 194
  venous return, 214
Cardiopulmonary exercise test, 56, 237
Central sleep apnea, 31, 331
Centriacinar emphysema, 63, *66*, 93, 226
Chest wall
  disease
    ankylosing spondylitis, 115–116
    scoliosis, 115
  elastic properties, pneumothorax, 112,
    112
  pressure-volume curve, *46*
Chronic bronchitis
  airway resistance, 48
  histologic changes, *69*
  pathogenesis, 68
  pathology, 68, *69*, *70*
Chronic obstructive pulmonary disease
    (COPD)
  acid–base status, 41, 224
  arterial blood gas, 236
  chronic bronchitis
    histologic changes, *69*
    pathogenesis, 68
    pathology, 68, *69*, *70*
  clinical features
    blue bloaters, 72, 74
    pink puffers, 70, *71–72*
  emphysema
    α_1-antitrypsin deficiency, 66, *67*
    centriacinar emphysema, 63, *66*
    clinical characteristics, 63
    microscopic appearance, 63, *64*
    panacinar emphysema, 63, *66*
    pathogenesis, 66, 68
    pathology, 63, *65*
    structural changes, 63, *65*
    topographic distribution of, *67*
  expiratory flow-volume curve, 11, *11*
  hypoxemia, 94, 226

  pulmonary function
    changes in early disease, 80–81
    control of ventilation, 80, *80*
    gas exchange, 76–79, *77*, *78*
    lung volume reduction surgery, 81
    pulmonary circulation, 79
    treatment of patients with, 81
    ventilatory capacity and mechanics,
      74–76
Cigarette smoking, 149
  airway conductance, 47, *48*
  carboxyhemoglobin level, 168, 231
  emphysema, 66
Closing volume, 14–15, 223
Coagulation, 132
Coal workers' pneumoconiosis, 155–156
Coccidiomycosis, 162, 163
Collagen vascular diseases, 111
Compliance, 46
Constant-volume ventilators, 206, *206*
Continuous positive airway pressure
    (CPAP), 31, 209
Cor pulmonale, 141, 230
Cough, 128
Cromolyn, 86
Cryptococcus, 163
Cystic fibrosis, 164–166, 232
Cystic fibrosis transmembrane regulator
    (CFTR), 239

D

Decompression sickness, 197
Desquamation, 100–101
Diaphragm
  emphysema, *72*
  respiratory failure, 177–178
Diaphragm fatigue, 177–178
Diffuse interstitial pulmonary fibrosis
  arterial hypoxemia, 118, 233
  clinical features, 101, *102*, *103*, 227
  diffusing capacity, carbon monoxide, 228
  maximal expiratory flow rate, 118, 228
  pathogenesis, 101
  pathology, 100–101, *100*
  pulmonary function, 118, 228
    control of ventilation, 107
    exercise, 106–107
    gas exchange, 103–106
    ventilatory capacity and mechanics,
      101–103
  treatment and outcomes, 107–108

Diffusing capacity, 41, 224
  doubling, 38, 224
  interpretation of, 38
  measurement of, 37, *37*
  reduced, 37–38
Diffusion
  aerosol deposition, 152
  Fick equation, 194
Diffusion impairment, 24–26, *25*
2,3-Diphosphoglycerate (DPG), *21*, 22, 224
Dynamic compression of airways, 8
  expiratory flow-volume curve, 7–8, *8*
  flow-volume curve, 10, *10*
  inspiratory flow-volume curve, 11, *12*
Dyspnea, 16, 52–53, 117, 128, 230, 238

E

Early airway disease tests, 15–16
Elastic recoil, 46, 75, *76*
Elastin, 99
Emphysema
  airway caliber in, *103*
  airway resistance, 48
  α_1-antitrypsin deficiency, 67, 68, 93, 226
  centriacinar emphysema, 63, *66*
  clinical characteristics, 63
  microscopic appearance, 63, *64*
  panacinar emphysema, 63, *66*
  pathogenesis, 66, 68
  pathology, 63, *65*
  structural changes, 63, *65*
  topographic distribution of, *67*
End-capillary blood, 193
Epithelial cell, 97, *98*, 99
Exercise
  diffuse interstitial pulmonary fibrosis,
    106–107
  mitral stenosis, 57, 226
  test, 50–52
Expiratory flow-volume curve
  COPD, 11, *11*
  normal patterns, 8, *8*
  obstructive and restrictive patterns, 8, *8*

F

Fick equation, 194
Flow-volume curve, 10, *10*
Forced expiration
  airway compression, 8, *8*
  forced expiratory flow calculation, 6, *6*
  normal pattern, 4, *5*
  obstructive pattern, 4, *5*
  restrictive pattern, 4, *5*
  vital capacity, 6–7
Forced expiratory volume (FEV)
  bronchodilators efficacy, 5
  chronic obstructive pulmonary disease,
    5, 18, 74
  measurement, *4*
Forced vital capacity (FVC), 4, *5*, 16, 236
Functional residual capacity (FRC), 226, 237
  asthma, 88
  body plethysmograph, 45
  elastic recoil, 55
Fungal infections, 162–163

G

Gas exchange
  arterial blood gases
    arterial P_{CO_2}, 32–34, *33*, 202
    arterial pH, 34–36
    arterial P_{O_2}, 21, *21*, 202 (*see also*
      Hypoxemia)
  asthma, 89–91, *89*, *90*
  chronic obstructive pulmonary disease,
    76–79, *77*, *78*
  diffuse interstitial pulmonary fibrosis,
    103–106
  diffusing capacity
    interpretation of, 38
    measurement of, 37, *37*
    reduced, 37–38
  pulmonary edema, 129–130
  pulmonary embolism, 137, *138*
Gastrointestinal bleeding, 215, 217

H

Haldane effect, 198
Helium dilution technique, 226
Henderson-Hasselbalch equation, 34
High-altitude pulmonary edema (HAPE),
  127, *127*, 230
High-frequency ventilation, 209
Histoplasmosis, 162
Human immunodeficiency virus (HIV), 231
Hydrocarbons, 148
Hygiene hypothesis, 83
Hyperbaric oxygen therapy, 196–197
Hypercapnia
  management, 184
  respiratory failure, 176–177
Hyperinflation, 237

Hypersensitivity pneumonitis
  clinical features, 110
  pathology, 110
  pulmonary function, 111
  treatment, 111
Hyperventilation
  COPD, oxygen uptake, 80, *80*
  respiratory alkalosis, 36
Hypoventilation
  alveolar gas equation, 22
  alveolar ventilation equation, 23
  cardinal physiologic features, 22
  causes of, 23–24, *24*, 24t
  increased arterial P_{CO_2}, 32
Hypoxemia, 237. *See also* Tissue hypoxia
  causes of
    diffusion impairment, 24–26, *25*
    hypoventilation, 22–24
    ventilation–perfusion inequality,
      28–30, *29*
  management, 184
  mechanisms, 41, 224
  multiple inert gas elimination technique,
    137
  oxygen delivery to tissues, 32
  oxygen therapy
    diffusion impairment, 191
    hypoventilation, 190–191
    shunt, 193, *193*
    ventilation–perfusion inequality,
      191–192, *192*
  respiratory failure, 175–176
Hypoxia
  tissue, 175–176
  ventilatory response, 49

I

Idiopathic pulmonary arterial hypertension,
  140–141, *140*
Impaction, 149, *150*
Infant respiratory distress syndrome, 183, 233
Infectious diseases
  AIDS, 163
  fungal infections, 162–163
  pneumonia, 160–162
  tuberculosis, 162
Inspiratory flow-volume curve, 11, *12*, 17, 223
Inspiratory positive airway pressure (IPAP),
  208–209
Intermittent hypoxemia, 31–32
Interstitial emphysema, 215
Interstitial fibrosis, 228

Interstitial pulmonary edema, 123, *123*, 143,
  229
Interstitium, 99
Intrapleural pressure, 8
Invasive mechanical ventilation, 186, 206, *206*,
  216
Irritant receptors, 107, 129

J

J receptors, 52

K

Kerley B lines, 128

L

Lactic acidosis, 36
Left atrial pressure, 139
Legionella, 232
Leukotriene receptor antagonists, 87
5-Lipoxygenase inhibitors, 87
Localized airway obstruction, 91–92
Lung function test. *See* Pulmonary function
  test
Lung overinflation, *72*
Lung volumes
  FRC
    body plethysmograph, 45
    helium dilution, 88–89
    interpretation, 45
    measurement, 45
    spirometer, 45
Lungs
  blood–gas barrier
    edematous thickening, 129
    hypoxemia, 27
    reduced diffusing capacity, 37–38, 106
  blood–gas interface, 91
  elastic properties
    compliance, 46
    interpretation, 46–47, *47*
    measurement, 46, *46*
Lymphangitis carcinomatosa, 111

M

Macrophages, 97, 154–155
Masks, 195
Maximum flows, 11, *11*

Mechanical ventilation
    ARDS, 218
    initiation of mechanical ventilation, 207
    invasive, 206, *206*
    modes of, 207
        continuous positive airway pressure, 209
        high-frequency ventilation, 209
        pressure control, 208
        pressure support, 208–209
        volume control, 208
    noninvasive, 206–207
    physiologic effects
        arterial P_{CO_2} reduction, 210–213, *211, 212*
        arterial P_{O_2}, increase in, 213–214
        cardiac arrhythmia, 215
        mechanical problems, 215
        miscellaneous hazards, 215
        pneumothorax, 215
        venous return, effects on, 214–215
    positive end-expiratory pressure, 209–210
    tank ventilators, 207
Metabolic acidosis, 36
Metabolic alkalosis, 36
Methylxanthines, 87
6-Minute walk test (6MWT), 51
Mucociliary dysfunction, 232
Mucociliary system, 153–154, *154*, 168, 231
Mucus, 68

N

Nasal cannulas, 195
    vs. masks, 195, 203, 233
Nedocromil, 87
Neoplastic diseases, 158–160
Neuromuscular disorders, 116
Nicotine, 231
Nitrogen oxides, 148, 171
Noninvasive mechanical ventilation, 206–207
Noninvasive positive pressure ventilation, 218, 235

O

Obstructive diseases
    COPD (*see* Chronic obstructive pulmo-
        nary disease)
    expiratory flow-volume curve, 8, *8*
    forced expiratory volume, 4, *5*
    single-breath nitrogen test, 14
Obstructive sleep apnea, 31

Occupational asthma, 158
Omalizumab, 87
Ondine's curse, 24
Orthopnea, 128
Oxygen dissociation curve
    anchor points, 17–18, *17*
    carbon monoxide poisoning, 203, 233
Oxygen therapy
    hazards of
        atelectasis, 199–201, *200*
        carbon dioxide retention, 197–198
        oxygen toxicity, 198
        prematurity, retinopathy of, 201
    hypoxemia
        diffusion impairment, 191
        hypoventilation, 190–191
        shunt, 193, *193*
        ventilation–perfusion inequality,
            191–192, *192*
    oxygen administration
        domiciliary and portable oxygen, 197
        high-flow delivery systems, 196
        hyperbaric oxygen, 196–197
        masks, 195
        nasal cannulas, 195
        tents, 196
        transtracheal oxygen, 196
        ventilators, 196
Oxygen (O_2) toxicity, 152, 174, 198, 234

P

Panacinar emphysema, 63, *66*
Particulate matter, 148
Peripheral chemoreceptors, 36, 91
Photochemical oxidants, 148
Pickwickian syndrome, 23
Plethysmography, 226
Pleural effusion, 114–115
Pleural thickening, 115
Pneumoconiosis, 155–156
Pneumonia, 216, 232
    clinical features, 161–162, *161*
    pathology, 161
    pulmonary function, 162
Pneumothorax, 215
    clinical features, 228
    pulmonary function, 114
    spontaneous, 113
    tension, 113–114
Positive end-expiratory pressure (PEEP), 235,
        240, 241
    increase in arterial P_{O_2}, 213–214

mechanical ventilation with, 130, 209–210, *211*
Prematurity, retinopathy of, 201
Pressure–volume curve
  edema, 129
  lung elasticity, 46, *46*
  sarcoidosis, 109
Pulmonary acinus, 63
Pulmonary arteriovenous malformation, 141
Pulmonary artery pressure, 134
Pulmonary circulation
  chronic obstructive pulmonary disease, 79
  edema, 130–131
  embolism, 134, 136, *136*
Pulmonary edema, 143, 229
  alveolar filling, 144, 229
  clinical features, 128
  heroin overdose, 128
  high-altitude pulmonary edema, 127
  neurogenic, 128
  pathogenesis, 125t
    decreased colloid osmotic pressure, *127*
    decreased interstitial pressure, 126
    increased capillary hydrostatic pressure, *126–127*
    increased capillary permeability, 126
    reduced lymph drainage, 126
    uncertain etiology, 127–128, *127*
  pathophysiology, 121–124
  pulmonary function
    control of ventilation, 130
    gas exchange, 129–130
    mechanics, 129
    pulmonary circulation, 130–131
  stages of, *122, 124*, 143
Pulmonary embolism
  causes, 144, 229
  clinical features, 132–133, *135*
  pathogenesis, 131–132
  pulmonary function
    gas exchange, 137, *138*
    mechanics, 136–137
    pulmonary circulation, 134, 136, *136*
  risk factor, 238
Pulmonary function test
  airway resistance, 47–49
  bronchiectasis, 164
  byssinosis, 157–158
  cystic fibrosis, 165
  dyspnea, 52–53
  exercise test, 50–52
  limits and benefits, 54–55
  lung elasticity, 46–47, *46, 47*

pneumoconiosis, 155–156
pneumonia, 162
reference values, 220, 220t
regional differences, 53–54, *54*
silicosis, 156
static lung volumes, 45
ventilation control, 49–50
ventilatory capacity
  expiratory flow-volume curve, 7–10, *8, 9*
  factors limiting, 7, *7*
  flow-volume curve, 10, *10*
  forced expiratory flow, 6, *6*
  forced expiratory volume, 4–5, *4, 5*
  peak expiratory flow rate, 11
Pulmonary hypertension, 138–141

R

Radioactive xenon method, 53, *135*
Reid index, 68
Residual volume, 15
Respiratory acidosis, 34–35, *35*, 232, 236
Respiratory alkalosis, 36
Respiratory failure
  acidosis in, 177
  arterial blood gas patterns, 174, *174*
  diaphragm fatigue, 177–178
  hypercapnia, 176–177
  hypoxemia, 175–176
  management, 184–185
  respiratory acidosis, 186
  types of
    acute on chronic lung disease, 179–180
    acute overwhelming lung disease, 178–179
    acute respiratory distress syndrome, 180–183, *180*
    infant respiratory distress syndrome, 183
    neuromuscular disorders, 179
Restrictive diseases
  chest wall disease
    ankylosing spondylitis, 115–116
    scoliosis, 115
  expiratory flow-volume curve, 8, *8*
  forced expiratory volume, 5, *5*
  neuromuscular disorders, 116
  parenchymal restrictive disease
    asbestosis, 111
    collagen vascular diseases, 111
    diffuse interstitial pulmonary fibrosis
      (*see* Diffuse interstitial pulmonary fibrosis)
    hypersensitivity pneumonitis, 110–111

Restrictive diseases (*Continued*)
    lymphangitis carcinomatosa, 111
    sarcoidosis, 108–110
    pleural diseases
        pleural effusion, 114–115
        pleural thickening, 115
        pneumothorax, 112–114
    single-breath nitrogen test, 14
Retinopathy, of prematurity, 201

S

Sarcoidosis
    clinical features, 110
    pathogenesis, 108
    pathology, 108
    pulmonary function, 111
    treatment, 110
Scoliosis, 115
Sedimentation, 150–152, *151*
Shunt
    hypoxemia, 27–28, *27*, 193, *193*
    oxygen therapy, 193, *193*
Silicosis
    clinical features, 156
    pathology, 156
    pulmonary function, 156
Single-breath nitrogen test, 12–14, 17,
    18, 223
Smog, 167, 230
    nitrogen oxides, 171
Spirometer, 45
Starling equation, 121
Sulfur oxides, 148
Symbols, 219–220

T

Tank ventilators, 207
Tension pneumothorax, 113–114
Tissue hypoxia, 175–176
Total lung capacity (TLC)
    chronic obstructive pulmonary
        disease, 75
Total ventilation, 210
Tracheal obstruction, 91
    airway resistance, 49
Tracheostomy, 196
Tuberculosis, 162
Type II alveolar epithelial cells, 97,
    98, 99

U

Uneven ventilation
    closing volume, 14–15
    early airway disease detection, 15–16
    mechanisms, *14*
    single-breath nitrogen test, 12–14
Units, 220

V

Vascular diseases
    pulmonary edema (*see* Pulmonary
        edema)
    pulmonary embolism (*see* Pulmonary
        embolism)
Vascular obstruction, 139
Vascular resistance, pulmonary, 139
Vasoconstriction, 139
Venous return, 214–215
Venous thrombi, 131
Ventilation
    control of
        COPD, 80
        diffuse interstitial pulmonary fibrosis,
           107
        interpretation, 49–50
        measurement, 49
        pulmonary edema, 130
    mechanical (*see* Mechanical ventilation)
Ventilation–perfusion inequality
    alveolar gas equation, 30
    alveolar–arterial oxygen difference, 29
    chronic obstructive pulmonary
        disease, 76
    hypoxemia, 28, 191–192, *192*, 227
    hypoxic vasoconstriction, 78–79
    increased arterial P_{CO_2}, *33*, 33–34
    in normal patient, 30, *30*
    respiratory failure, 174
Ventilation–perfusion ratios
    ARDS, *182*, 183
    asthma, *89*
    atelectasis, 199–201, *200*
    chronic obstructive pulmonary disease,
        77, *77*
    in normal patient, 30, *30*
Ventilator-associated pneumonia, 215
Ventilator-induced lung injury, 215
Ventilators
    constant-volume ventilators, *206*
    tank ventilators, 207

Ventilatory capacity
  asthma, 87–89, *88*
  chronic obstructive pulmonary disease, 74–76
  diffuse interstitial pulmonary fibrosis, 101–103
  factors limiting, 7, *7*
  flow-volume curve
    dynamic compression of airways, 10, *10*
    maximum flows, 11, *11*
    forced expiratory flow, 6, *6*
    forced expiratory volume, 4–5, *4, 5*
    peak expiratory flow rate, 11
Virchow's triad, 131
Vital capacity, 6–7